TAMING

THE 7 MOST FATTENING EXCUSES IN THE WORLD

Re-thinking Your Healthy Obsession Pathway to Lifelong Weight Loss

DANIEL S. KIRSCHENBAUM, PH.D., ABPP

ISBN: 978-1-7323362-5-4

Edited by: Elizabeth Russell

Warren publishing

Published by Warren Publishing
Charlotte, NC
www.warrenpublishing.net
Printed in the United States

ACKNOWLEDGMENTS

First and foremost, I am especially grateful to the amazing artist who transformed my very rough linear sketches of the Stymie Beasts into the wonderfully expressive mini-dragon versions in this book: Sheila Macomber. Sheila also created some of the other illustrations in this book. We have worked together for more than thirty years and 100% of the time her creations yielded "Wow-Sheila!!!" moments (as you can see at her website: www.sheilamacomber.com).

The Stymie Beasts did not start out as they appear now, not by a long shot. Warren Publishing's Vice President and Editor-in-Chief Amy Trainor Ashby helped tremendously by encouraging Sheila and me to re-work our former more monstrous versions into the current cuter creatures. Amy and her colleague, Mindy Kuhn, President of Warren Publishing, supported this project vigorously from its inception, including Mindy's creative efforts that produced the beautiful cover and design of the book.

All of the twenty-two endorsers of this book who appear in its opening pages truly believe in the value of the scientifically based, empathic, and effective approach presented here. They have all witnessed its ability to help people succeed in one of the most challenging quests humans face: radically transforming their bodies despite the biological, cultural, and personal barriers that powerfully resist such changes. I sincerely thank each of them for their unwavering appreciation of this work, especially the remarkably supportive, superb clinician/advocate Sue Shrifter-Fialkow, MA, LCSW, the co-founder of our former twenty-plus-year practice in Chicago—Center for Behavioral Medicine.

Finally, I have been asked repeatedly to explain the source of the energy and drive that led to the creation of this book, my thirteenth, at this stage in my career (forty-three years after receiving my Ph.D.). Personal fitness, daily exercise, maintaining a healthy weight for fifty years, golf, bowling, jogging/walking, inspiring tunes, remarkable colleagues, brilliant, dedicated scientific predecessors—all come to mind. But, there is a simpler foundational essence in this case: love. I'm incredibly fortunate to feel that every minute of every day from my wife, Sue Payne, and from my wonderful millennial children: Alex, Max, and Rosie Kirschenbaum.

ENDORSEMENTS

"We strongly endorse Dr. Kirschenbaum's wonderful new book. Collectively, in our integrative healthcare pain management practice, with Dr. Kirschenbaum taking the lead on weight and stress/mood management, we have helped our patients lose substantial amounts of weight, feel happier, and experience much less chronic pain. Some of these patients could not walk; some used canes initially and then kicked those canes into recycling bins as they got thinner and stronger. Dr. Kirschenbaum's compassionate and scientifically grounded approach helps people re-route their thinking to tame unfortunate cognitive barriers and very comfortably develop life-changing healthy obsessions."

–GEORGIA PAIN AND SPINE CARE, NEWNAN, GEORGIA:
R. CHARLES BROWNLOW, MD, CEO, LA'SHUNN DOGGETTE, NP,
ALI KASSAMALI, MD, ASHLEY MILLER, NP, KENT REMLEY, MD,
SANDEEP VAID, MD, JAY RICE, ATC, CHIEF OPERATING OFFICER,
TYLER SNOW, ATC, DIRECTOR OF CLINICAL OPERATIONS

"As Dr. Kirschenbaum continues to be a wise guiding light in helping all scientists understand the complex medical, cognitive-behavioral, and emotional challenges of weight management, his books for the public are profound, pragmatic, and personable. I can find no better compendium of facts and clear practical advice for overweight people than this one. The value to all who read Taming the 7 Most Fattening Excuses… will be self-evident from the very first chapter. I have no doubt that this book will be used as a reference book for effective weight control for decades to come. No wonder countless obesity experts entrust their patients to Dr. Kirschenbaum."

–JOHN RABKIN, MD, DIRECTOR, PACIFIC LAPAROSCOPY, SAN FRANCISCO,
CALIFORNIA; FELLOW, AMERICAN COLLEGE OF SURGERY

"Taming the 7 Most Fattening Excuses... *is a wonderfully written, elegantly simplified, and compassionate approach to healthy weight loss! No more old excuses and failed attempts! Dr. Kirschenbaum makes weight loss and maintenance attainable with practical explanations, a wonderful new method to re-configure unfortunate ways of thinking into constructive actions, and a holistic sensibility that incorporates the essential elements of long-term success. I've witnessed Dr. Kirschenbaum's approach become a powerful, life-changing program for dozens of weight controllers—truly transformative in understanding our relationships with the way we think, behave, and maximize our health and well-being!"*

–SONIA SAMPAT, PSYD, CHICAGO, ILLINOIS,
FORMER WELLSPRING WISCONSIN CAMP CLINICAL DIRECTOR

"As a physician, author, and health coach, I am acutely aware of the complexity of the science of weight management. That made me deeply excited to read Dr. Kirschenbaum's Taming the 7 Most Fattening Excuses.... *Dr. Kirschenbaum translated the science of weight management and decision making into a very clearly focused and well-written book. Now, thousands (millions?) of weight controllers can see how to neutralize obstructive cognitive biases to re-route their thinking and implement the very effective VLF HOP approach—and permanently change their language from can't to can."*

–DR. PETER NIEMAN, FRCP, FAAP CALGARY WEIGHT MANAGEMENT CENTRE;
UNIVERSITY OF CALGARY; PRESIDENT, ALBERTA CHAPTER OF THE AMERICAN
ACADEMY OF PEDIATRICS; AUTHOR OF MOVING FORWARD

"At last, a scientifically grounded, practical guide to effective and safe long-term weight loss. Taming the 7 Most Fattening Excuses... *will help weight controllers re-think their approach and perhaps 'stop the insanity' of believing that low-carb, gluten free, and anti-all processed foods (no yogurt or veggie burgers, really?) hold the 'secrets' to losing weight. Dr. Kirschenbaum has been a distinguished researcher, master therapist, and consultant for forty years, focused on weight management. He has helped thousands of people lose weight and feel better permanently."*

–ROB SMITH, PHD, CERTIFIED MENTAL PERFORMANCE
CONSULTANT, ASSOCIATION FOR APPLIED SPORT PSYCHOLOGY;
CLINICAL PSYCHOLOGIST, WALTHAM, MASSACHUSETTS

"Dr. Kirschenbaum's strategies for 'taming the beasts within'—our negative attitudes, excuses, self-defeating thoughts —provide an essential component of effective lifelong weight loss. His plan is based on his many decades of helping people turn their lives around by losing weight with sustainable lifestyle adaptations. Backed by scientific research, his key steps include: restructured thinking or 'turn-around-talk,' healthy eating, and consistent exercise. Those struggling with weight, as well as health professionals, will find this book refreshing, insightful, helpful, and most of all—effective!"

–GEORGIA KOSTAS, MPH, RDN, LD, AUTHOR,
THE COOPER CLINIC SOLUTION TO THE DIET REVOLUTION, FORMER
DIRECTOR AND FOUNDER OF THE COOPER CLINIC NUTRITION
PROGRAM AT THE COOPER AEROBICS CENTER, DALLAS, TX

"It has been an honor and pleasure to work with Dr. Kirschenbaum for many years and learn from his incredible expertise. Our research comparing exceptionally successful to unsuccessful weight controllers verified Dr. Kirschenbaum's previous findings about the major contributors to success, including the vital roles of consistent self-monitoring and healthy obsessions. We also discovered that broadening sources of motivation may improve weight management; for example, focusing on not only prior triumphs, but also memories of frustrations and emotional challenges caused by excess weight. In his fantastic and very important new book, Taming the 7 Most Fattening Excuses..., Dr. Kirschenbaum shows not only how problematic decision making creates Stymie Beasts, but also how to transform those cognitive barriers into positive action. Just as his research and programs have helped thousands enjoy more health and happiness, this book could help many more thousands dramatically improve the quality of their lives."

–KRISTEN CARAHER, PSYD, ASSISTANT PROFESSOR OF PSYCHIATRY,
UNIVERSITY OF IOWA CARVER COLLEGE OF MEDICINE

"During my time as Director of a United Kingdom-based weight loss camp, I worked with an incredibly diverse range of students from all over the Middle East and Europe. My colleagues and I helped to implement Dr. Kirschenbaum's approach, and the campers and families embraced it, despite its radical departure from their usual routines in both eating and moving. The new material in his latest book, particularly the Stymie Beasts, will add even greater understanding to the best approach to long-term weight loss and lifestyle change."

–JENNI HUME, CAMPAIGN MANAGER,
THE ASSOCIATION FOR THE PROTECTION OF
RURAL SCOTLAND, EDINBURGH, SCOTLAND,
FORMER WELLSPRING UK CAMP DIRECTOR

"*Dr. Kirschenbaum's* Taming the 7 Most Fattening Excuses... *will undoubtedly become the bible of cognitive challenges and solutions in the quest for permanent weight management. This thoroughly engaging, hands-on book will engender new and truly refreshing hope for readers, based on solid science and decades of remarkably successful clinical experience with literally thousands of grateful participants. Weight controllers can truly follow the clear pathway Dr. Kirschenbaum provides to finally achieve transformative lifestyle change.*"
–Susan Shrifter-Fialkow, MA, LCSW, Chicago, IL

"*Dr. Kirschenbaum's book,* Taming the 7 Most Fattening Excuses..., *uses his expertise in psychological and biological science to show weight controllers how to overcome self-defeating thinking and behaving via new understanding, work, and persistence. Dr. Kirschenbaum's book is based on his decades of experience and scientific research, yet his writing is remarkably straightforward, funny, and approachable. I highly recommend this book to anyone who has been frustrated by weight-loss fads and is ready for a scientifically-based, effective approach to achieve a healthy weight and lifestyle—and tremendous personal satisfaction for mastering such a difficult challenge.*"
–Ross Krawczyk, PhD, Licensed Clinical Psychologist, Assistant Professor of Psychology, The College of St. Rose, Albany, New York

"*With* Taming the 7 Most Fattening Excuses..., *Dr. Daniel Kirschenbaum continues in his role as the foremost author of communicating the science plus the 'how to' of weight loss. Taming... is perfect for healthcare professionals and their patients, as well as for consumers too smart to succumb to the promise of the latest fad diet. It's written in user-friendly language, based on the most recent research in the scientific study of obesity. What really sets this book apart, though, is that Dr. Kirschenbaum uses a cognitive behavioral framework in the form of 'Stymie Beasts' to humanize the familiar stumbling blocks of long-suffering dieters. He also provides the 'how to' tools to 'tame the beasts;' that is, to make the elusive transition from 'I can't do it' to 'I can do it,' and achieve lasting weight management. These tools, along with his empathetic approach to enhance motivation, will make* Taming... *an invaluable resource to use with our patients. Bravo!*"
–Lisa Murphy, LCSW & William Hartman, Ph.D., San Francisco, California

"Dr. Kirschenbaum has distilled the science of long-term weight control into this logical program that works! As a child and family therapist, I especially love the cognitive behavioral components and have seen firsthand how Dr. Kirschenbaum's scientific holistic approach allows weight controllers to overcome and master their automatic thoughts, motivational hurdles, and misconceptions about what it takes to be successful for a lifetime. The straightforward and accessible format helps my clients get right to work: aiming for clearly-defined targets, monitoring and measuring progress, and discovering creative ways to make modifications that allow them to enjoy their journey in sustainable ways. After a lifetime dedicated to understanding the psychology of weight control, Dr. Kirschenbaum has cultivated a program that is a beacon of hope in this bariatric age."
–HEATHER RUTH RICHARDSON, LPC, BREVARD, NORTH CAROLINA

"I worked with Dr. Kirschenbaum for seven years at Wellspring weight loss camps where he was the Chief Program Officer (designer of the approach), Clinical Director, and eventually President of Wellspring. I witnessed dramatic transformations in hundreds of young people when they followed his weight loss plan. Campers lost an average of four lbs. a week, really enjoyed the food, and didn't feel deprived or hungry. Many returned year after year to keep making progress on developing their commitments and healthy obsessions—and to continue losing weight. In this excellent new book, Dr. Kirschenbaum writes about re-routing thinking to promote the use of scientifically based approaches rather than giving up or continuing to try useless fad diets."
–WILL BETTMANN, MA, JD, ASSISTANT PRINCIPAL,
CHAPEL HILL/CARRBORO SCHOOL DISTRICT, NORTH CAROLINA,
FORMER WELLSPRING NEW YORK CAMP DIRECTOR

"Dr. Kirschenbaum tackles one of the most challenging aspects of weight loss—the mental battle. He breaks it down in a well-researched, scientific approach that demystifies the mental barriers to weight loss and offers a straightforward program that works. This book is a wealth of information from a lifetime very successful weight controller and scientist who has helped countless individuals reach a healthy weight and maintain it!"
–SUSAN KIRK EdD, LCSW, MARSHALL, NORTH CAROLINA

TABLE OF CONTENTS

PART I: Understanding and Taming the Cognitive Barriers (Seven Stymie Beasts)

PART II: The VLF* Healthy Obsession Pathway (HOP*) in Five Steps

PART I

Understanding and Taming the Cognitive Barriers (Seven Stymie Beasts)

CHAPTER 1
Introduction

"I can't lose weight. I've tried everything; I'm just tired of the roller coaster—lose weight, feel great gain it all back and then some, and feel like crap. I've tried every diet and program; nothing works for me. I'm done."

Does this quote ring any bells for you? Many weight controllers find this sentiment very familiar, and certainly understandable. It hurts to keep putting so much effort into such an important quest without substantial payoff. If you tried to lose weight and repeatedly lost and regained the weight, then you would undoubtedly feel disappointment. You might become disappointed in both yourself and the book or program or approach you used. You might also dislike the negative reactions of those around you to such failures.

Some people turn their disappointment into a powerful barrier against change. That barrier starts life as an excuse, essentially an explanation for such failures. Excuses can protect our views of ourselves as good, competent people. For example, if I decide that I *cannot* lose weight, then I can forgive myself for failing to lose weight despite joining Weight Watchers or using Slim Fast for several weeks. After all, how can I expect myself to succeed at something I fundamentally cannot do?

Psychologist Barry Schlenker and his colleagues described excuses in this way: Excuses can keep us from getting mad at ourselves, protecting us from viewing ourselves in a negative light. Excuses can also manage others' impressions of us. If we excuse ourselves by saying we cannot lose weight, then that resolves the conflict about living with excess weight. We take ourselves out of the conflict by giving up on further attempts to try to make it happen. When a spouse nudges the "cannot do it" decision-maker to go for it again, that person just invokes the excuse, "I would try it again except I now know that I *cannot* do it." Some following this path might say to their spouses, "You saw how hard I worked at X, Y, and Z weight-loss programs/diets, right? Well, I just cannot do it again."

Excuses as Stymie Beasts

I view a decision like *I cannot lose weight* as something much more alive and dynamic than just an excuse. To breathe life into such excuses, I decided to animate them—creating anthropomorphisms called Stymie Beasts. If you can start viewing problematic excuses as beasts, you can start battling them. After all, psychologists view excuses as primarily protective devices allowing us to view ourselves as good people. In order to shake off that unfortunate protective coating that excuses provide, let's try placing those decisions outside of ourselves—as Stymie Beasts that we can fight—and defeat.

In a nutshell, these two points summarize the value of creating Stymie Beasts when trying to overcome the internal challenge that excuses impose:

- **Empathic, Not Negative:** If people didn't face a major struggle when trying to lose weight permanently, the fifty- to one-hundred-billion-dollar diet industry would just fade away. Instead of feeling blamed when reading this book about excuses, I hope you will see that I very much appreciate the remarkable difficulty of this quest. I blame you not at all for excusing ineffective ways of pursuing permanent weight loss. I just want to help you find better solutions to this difficult problem. I also know that people often react to negative feedback by rejecting the source of the feedback. Let's not let that happen here.

- **External, Less Internal:** Psychologist Craig Anderson and his colleagues from the University of Missouri reviewed research that showed blaming yourself for difficulties in life can decrease motivation to change. For example, Sally used to say to herself, "I'm pathetic for not losing weight." What's a good way for Sally to avoid feeling pathetic? Decreasing efforts (motivation) to lose weight would get her to feel less bothered by this part of her life. In other words, if she avoids trying to lose weight, she can focus her attention on other aspects of her life— with resulting fewer negative self-condemnations.

  In contrast, attributing responsibility for one's difficulties to more external sources can help keep you more motivated to change. So, trying to tame a Stymie Beast might make the process of modifying excuses much easier than blaming yourself.

What is a "stymie?" A stymie in golf happens when an opponent's ball gets between the golfer's ball and the hole on the green. Golfers wrote the original rules of golf in 1744, but then golfers from a more modern era changed the stymie rule two centuries later, in 1952. Before the 1952 change, golfers sometimes found themselves blocked from the goal of getting their golf balls into the hole when putting because they were stymied by their opponent. The stymie in golf required golfers during those two centuries to try to putt around the stymie ball or chip over it to get to the hole. Since the rule change in 1952, an opponent's golf ball that stymies yours now simply gets marked by a coin. The coin is moved if necessary so that nothing blocks the golfer from putting directly toward the hole.

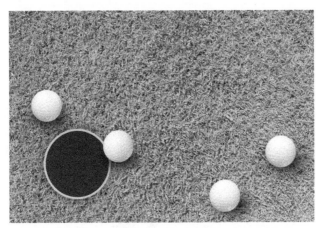

Dictionary.com defines stymie more broadly than its origins in the game of golf. That definition describes stymies as *barriers that thwart efforts to resolve problems.* The barriers can emerge as giant walls with barbed wire on top, making them seem almost insurmountable. But Stymie Beasts create barriers that we can shrink into mere annoyances, despite their desire to oppose constructive progress.

gut brain?

Here's what the *I Can't Do It* Stymie Beast looks like:

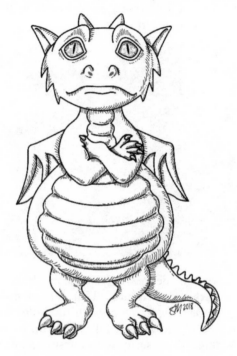

This "Can't" Stymie Beast visually represents a type of decision: a harmful excuse that resists persistent efforts to change for the good. This Beast can create a powerful barrier between you and a better life.

You can begin to overcome these excuses by first embracing them as Beasts. Instead of accepting this type of thought as part of you (partly defining who you are), try thinking of those excuses as something external to you—out there, staring at you, making your life more difficult: a cognitive challenge to you. This Can't Stymie Beast has six kindred spirits (six other Beasts) that you will come to know in this book. These Beasts create major obstacles to incredibly important goals in your life. Those goals can include vastly improved health, improved fitness, a positive sense of personal pride and power, and the success that all successful weight controllers experience every day.

THE ORIGIN OF STYMIE BEASTS: COGNITIVE BIASES

Accepting the existence of Stymie Beasts allows you to begin to take steps to tame them. Perhaps you will accept them even more once you understand their origins. For example, the Can't Stymie Beast comes from repeated failures to lose weight. But does that really make sense? Remember the famous Thomas Edison quote about his two thousand failures to create the light bulb? He argued that those were not failures at all. Every one of them revealed to him and his colleagues exactly how *not* to make a lightbulb. In other words, he translated those experiences into successes through a process of learning how to succeed. Another related quote comes from one of the greatest baseball players of all time, Willie Mays. When asked how he got so lucky to be so fantastic at baseball, he quipped (very wisely), "The harder I work, the luckier I get."

Translating failures into Can't means you do *not* use Edison's or Mays' perspective when pursuing your goal of permanent weight loss. Once you firmly plant your decision about losing weight into the Can't world, you agree to accept your life, and your weight, just as it is, never again striving to achieve an important goal. Why do that?

Consider the alternative to the *I Can't Do It* rationale for discontinuing efforts to lose weight by a very overweight person. One of my clients, Bob, tried numerous methods to lose weight and kept regaining the weight over a period of twenty years. Then, he decided to do some research to find the best approach available to him. He discovered that many people, just like him, try various commercially advertised programs and buy the latest diet books. The scientific literature (as translated by Consumer Reports and in the published recommendations of expert groups, like the US Preventive Services Task Force) shows that diets generally fail, reading books on weight loss (sometimes called bibliotherapy) almost never works, and research on commercial programs like the ones he tried show them to fail almost all of the time.

On the other hand, the research evidence shows that Cognitive Behavior Therapy (CBT) provided by licensed providers (primarily psychologists) can help most people most of the time. So, Bob found me (a CBT specialist focused on weight management) and, lo and behold, he then successfully lost sixty pounds and maintained that loss for years afterwards. Despite the possibility of this alternative to the Can't Beast, many people let such Stymie Beasts determine their thinking and behaviors. This decision causes them to stop all efforts to achieve such important goals as weight reduction and improved fitness.

The creation of these oftentimes powerful Stymie Beasts starts with a very common tendency to make unfortunate decisions. That tendency uses biased methods of decision-making called *cognitive biases*. Psychologists Herbert Simon, Daniel Kahneman, Amos Tversky, and many others devoted much of their lives to studying these biases. They conducted dozens of important studies that showed us the very nature and power of these cognitive biases, beautifully summarized in the best seller by the 2002 Noble Laureate, Princeton University Professor Daniel Kahneman, *Thinking Fast and Slow*. We now know that we often make decisions without examining the pros and cons, the scientific evidence, or other super-rational means (like looking for high-quality information vs. accepting the top organic results from an online search).

For an example of the way someone can create a Stymie Beast, consider what some overweight people do when they decide that their efforts don't just represent a particular book or program; instead these folks decide that those efforts represent *all* possible ways to lose weight. Clearly, this kind of decision, a cognitive bias, distorts reality— ignoring scientific evidence about what really works to help people lose weight. In other words, cognitive biases promote decision making based on something other than a systematic analysis of all the facts. Table 1-1 presents a list of ten cognitive biases that definitely affect weight controllers:

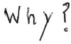 Why?

Ten Cognitive Biases

Affect	Making choices based on **feelings** more than analysis: "The emotional tail wags the rational dog."
Anchoring	**First** piece of information becomes more important than anything else.
Availability	**WYSIATI**–What You See Is All There Is: Gives great power to commercials, dominant ideas or programs readily available.
Confirmation	Seeking and attending primarily/only to information that **conforms** with our existing way of thinking about something.
Conservation	Favoring **current** approaches despite new evidence favoring new or different approaches; resistence to shifting paradigms.
Innovation	The opposite of conservatism: Favoring something just because it's **new,** not because the evidence suggests it's better than current approaches.
Outcome	Basing decisions on **outcomes** regardless of how the outcome was achieved (luck > science, logic).
Overconfidence	Over-valuing our impulses or instinctive beliefs or **guesses;** expecting our ideas to work out right regardless of the actual challenges we face; viewing our ideas through very rose-colored glasses.
Recency	Focusing on and remembering the **latest** information, what was heard or experienced more recently, more than information or experiences from earlier times.
Representative	Greatly exaggerating the commonness of something just based on **experiencing** it or seeing it, rather than relying on base rate statistics or systematic analysis of the quality of information.

TABLE 1-1

Which of these ten cognitive biases helps breathe life into the *I Can't Do It* Stymie Beast? Several possibilities exist to answer that question. In my view, Availability and Representative biases often operate for those who develop Can't Beasts. Let's say a weight controller saw lots of commercials for a famous support group program focused on counting calories as points and another very famous low-carb diet book. Then, that person tried both approaches several times each over a three-year period. As is the case for most people who try such approaches, they failed. The person may have lost some weight in both efforts, but that weight returned rather quickly and possibly increased. Those two readily available approaches impacted this weight controller. The failure to achieve lasting success may also have resulted in a conclusion focused on the self: I can't do this. That conclusion makes the false assumption that other (better) approaches do not exist, in part because other approaches are not nearly as available to that weight controller (Availability Bias). Some of those other approaches also have far more science behind them (as you will see in Chapters 5-8). This means that a false and destructive conclusion emerged based on a Representative Bias—the view that failure at two approaches accurately represents that person's fundamental inability to succeed using any other approach.

In this book, you will come to understand, in depth, the nature of these cognitive biases. You will learn about the ten most common ones listed in Table 1-1, all of which produce and nurture seven Stymie Beasts like the Can't Beast. Here's why that matters:

You cannot tame what you cannot see.

Once you see the enemy for what it is, you can learn how to defeat it.

How Taming Stymie Beasts
Can Help You Lose Weight

We mentioned that viewing excuses as external to you can help you overcome such self-defeating decisions. Let's consider an example to help you understand and appreciate this viewpoint: perfectionism.

Psychologist Randy Frost and his colleagues and students at Smith College have studied perfectionism more than any other researchers. Dr. Frost defined this personality quality as the tendency to set very high standards and to evaluate oneself in overly critical ways. To judge if you lean in this direction, answer the following three questions derived from Dr. Frost and colleagues' Multidimensional Perfectionism Scale, using a 1 (Strongly Disagree) to 5 (Strongly Agree) rating scale:

_____ If I fail at work or school, I am a failure as a person.

_____ If I fail partly, it is as bad as being a complete failure.

_____ If someone does a task better than me, then I feel like I failed.

If you strongly agreed with these three assertions (rated them with fours and fives), then you're leaning in a perfectionistic direction. Notice how these questions suggest that problems with performance translate directly to problems with yourself as a person. Fortunately, these rather extreme reactions can change, especially by using an approach created in the 1950s by the well-known psychologist, Dr. Albert Ellis, that he called Rational Emotive Therapy (RET).

RET, something you will learn more about in Chapter 3, is an important technique within the broader scientifically based approach to helping people change called Cognitive Behavior Therapy (CBT). RET helps people change often exaggerated negative self-talk to a more balanced positive approach. For example, instead of saying that failing partly means failing as a person, RET suggests that failing partly may not be ideal, but it says virtually nothing about your personal qualities or overall success as a person. Dr. Frost and colleagues demonstrated that using RET to reverse these exaggerated negative beliefs about oneself greatly reduced perfectionism and improved moods.

Here's a poem I wrote—designed to reduce the power of the Can't Beast using RET principles. In this case, RET principles help change "can't" to "can." It changes the language of the beastly barrier to persistence, making that "can't" decision into something far more intentional. As you read it, see if you recognize more leverage to change caused by this rather simple change in language:

WITH WON'TS, YOU CAN'T

If you can't run every morning,
Then you can run in the evening.
If you can't run,
Then you can walk briskly.
If you can't walk briskly,
Then you can just walk slowly or
*   treadmill or bike or swim.*
If you can't do any of this,
Then, let's face it,
You can't only because you won't.
You can't walk,
Because you won't make it matter enough.
You can succeed by changing can'ts to cans,
But not with won'ts.
Can you make yourself matter every day?

So, let's talk Stymie Beasts now. What's the connection? The Can't Beast believes that past failures doom all future efforts. Failure, in this case, leads to views of oneself as a total failure at weight management—forever. Some perfectionists view almost any failure as a justification (excuse) for viewing oneself as a total failure as a person. Just because you didn't win a tennis match or struggled to pass a test at school, does that really mean you're a failure as a human being? Aren't all people allowed to struggle at least sometimes—and still succeed overall as human beings? I bet you know at least several incredibly successful people; not one of them succeeded at every test and endeavor.

Viewing challenges as coming from a force other than yourself can take some of the power from these problematic excuses. The Stymie Beasts allow you to separate those excuses from your sense of self. You can learn to view your excuses as part of a process of understanding your world, not a means to define, much less condemn, you as a person. You can stare those decisions (Stymie Beasts) in the face and make different choices. That process can free you up to pursue the challenging goal of permanent weight control. That's exactly what RET does for perfectionists—changes their thinking about failures to make them more okay, more a part of life—events that can teach us something. This works far better than using failures at specific tasks to condemn our very selves.

In this book, you will learn RET thinking to help you manage your Stymie Beasts, just as perfectionists learn to modify their thinking. Perfectionists use RET to get beyond momentary setbacks by viewing themselves as okay despite such failures at specific events. You can learn to defeat problematic thinking and get beyond that barrier to your own success. By carefully reading this book, you can allow yourself to succeed at weight control.

The three keys to success presented in this book are:

1. How to recognize and understand COGNITIVE BIASES—the unfortunate (but very common) ways of thinking that sustain your Stymie Beast.

2. How to tame your Stymie Beast by using two very effective strategies:
   - Therapeutic Understanding of Science (TUS)— how to use science to make better informed and more effective decisions; and
   - Rational Emotive Therapy (RET)—how to change the internal dialogues you use to think more calmly and clearly to defeat your Stymie Beasts.
3. After taming these Beasts, you will become truly ready to lose weight permanently by using the VLF Healthy Obsession Pathway (HOP), following five steps to get there:
   - Learn what really causes weight problems
   - Develop a HEALTHY OBSESSION
   - Follow a Very Low Fat (VLF) eating plan (assisted by two other major dietary principles to decrease appetite deliciously and effectively—Low Caloric Density and Caloric Control)
   - Maximize movement
   - Enhance support from others and your environment

PREVIEW OF A SUMMARY OF HOW TO TAME YOUR STYMIE BEASTS

In the next two chapters, you will learn first how Stymie Beasts emerge from biases that impact decision making. Then you will discover two powerful ways to tame such challenged ways of making decisions. As a hint of things to come, please review this table (from the end of Chapter 3) that summarizes this fascinating information—as a way to start considering your own barriers to success:

SUMMARY OF STYMIE BEASTS AND KEY TAMING THOUGHTS

Stymie Beasts	Stymie Thoughts	Taming Thoughts
	CAN'T: I've tried every diet, and nothing works for me. I'm done!	Just because you have not succeeded so far, that does not mean you cannot find a new way to lose weight. You have not yet tried the type of cognitive behavior therapy approach (VLF HOP's five steps) featured in this book. You can do this, if you give science a real chance to help you.
	ADDICT: I just can't get past my addiction to food.	Food addiction is more myth than reality. You're just finding it tough to avoid certain problematic foods—and to succeed at the substantial challenge of weight control.
	HATE: There's nothing I hate more than exercising; well, maybe dieting.	You can find plenty of lovable foods that work great on this program. You can also learn to enjoy the many benefits of movement, without training for a marathon. Achieving some success will help quiet the hate.
	LAZY: I know it would be good to lose weight, but I'm just too lazy.	The CBT program in this book makes losing weight easier and more achievable. Success will energize you; you can use that energy to strive toward even more success.

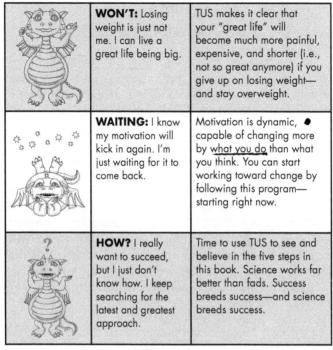

	WON'T: Losing weight is just not me. I can live a great life being big.	TUS makes it clear that your "great life" will become much more painful, expensive, and shorter (i.e., not so great anymore) if you give up on losing weight—and stay overweight.
	WAITING: I know my motivation will kick in again. I'm just waiting for it to come back.	Motivation is dynamic, capable of changing more by what you do than what you think. You can start working toward change by following this program—starting right now.
	HOW? I really want to succeed, but I just don't know how. I keep searching for the latest and greatest approach.	Time to use TUS to see and believe in the five steps in this book. Science works far better than fads. Success breeds success—and science breeds success.

TABLE 3-3

Bringing HOP to Life:
Three Amazing Case Studies

In the rest of this book, you will read plenty of information based on science, including graphs showing remarkably good results for the Healthy Obsession Pathway, or HOP. Learning about real people who used this approach successfully might increase your excitement about HOP, almost certainly more than hearing about the numbers. The following three stories include three very different people who transformed themselves using HOP. In these cases, these people accomplished major lifestyle changes with the considerable assistance of professionally conducted programs. Still, these fine folks have nurtured and elaborated their healthy obsessions enough to win their battles with their powerful biological resistance in the face of an antagonistic obesogenic culture for many years.

Can you find some inspiration in their stories? If they can do it, can you?

STEVE M.

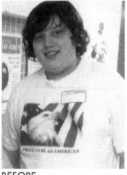 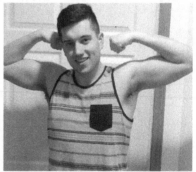

BEFORE:
12 years old 5'5"188 lbs.

NOW (8 years later): 20 years old 6'2" 200 lbs: 9 inches taller, much stronger (more muscular), and just 12 lbs. heavier; pitcher and first baseman and captain of his team—a junior at Ferris State University in Michigan

Three years after Steve attended a Wellspring camp, his very dedicated and loving father, Dave, wrote to me to help inspire others, including the employees at Wellspring. After presenting the exchanges between Dave and me, I will present Steve's own view of his current life—four-plus years after the exchange between Dave and me about Steve and their family's transformation.

Letters from a Father about His Son's and Family's Remarkable 3.5 Year Weight-loss Journey

12/5/13

Dear Dan,

It has been three and a half years since Steve attended camp. I wanted to share with you his story. When Steve arrived at camp, he was twelve years old, 5' 4.5" tall, and weighed 187.6 pounds. He lost 19.4 pounds in four weeks at Wellspring Pennsylvania. Today, he is 16 and stands 6' 1" and weighs 160 pounds. I don't normally take the time to do stuff like this, especially three years later when most people may not remember Steve. But, I thought it was important.

Four years ago, Steve was the "fat kid" that no one wanted on their team; other kids would make fun of him on the ice during hockey, and he was the slowest kid on the baseball team. That has all changed.[Wellspring's approach] has changed his life. He has improved at all the sports he plays. He played travel baseball last year and is still in hockey. He was the fourth leading scorer on his team last year and scored more goals last year than all of his other years combined. He is also continuing his baseball and has become one of the best hitters. He is still on plan, he eats well, and never strays; he has incredible will power, even when temptation surrounds him. I want to thank all of you from the bottom of my heart. I would do it all over again, but fortunately I do not have to.

Sincerely,
    Dave M

12/6/13

Dear Dave,
    Thanks so much for sharing the wonderful news about Steve with us. We're hoping that you might be willing to say even more about what your family did to support him so remarkably well over these past 3.5 years.

    Thanks again, Dan Kirschenbaum

12/11/13

Dear Dan,
    Sure. I can say a great deal about Steve's progress and our family's support of him over these past several years.
    Steve was always a heavy kid. I did not think that his diet was all that unhealthy; however, he continued to gain weight as he got older. We became very concerned that he was approaching a very unhealthy size. I was also worried about his potential life span carrying that much weight and about the seemingly free pass people get for making fun of the fat kid. Even though he had lots of friends, you can always hear the mockery from the outside.
    My wife and I obviously did not have the tools needed to help him and made the decision to do something about it. My main concern was that Steve would be starved for four weeks and then run like a dog at your weight loss camp. He'd then lose a bunch of weight at camp, only to put

it back on when he returned home. So I was really worried after we dropped him off for his four weeks of camp.

On his first call home, I only had two questions for him. Are you ever hungry and are they making you exercise too much? He told me that he was never hungry and that there was always enough food to eat. That made me very happy and helped to allay some of my fears. He also told me that he loved all of the activities. Even though he was heavy, he always liked sports and activity was not the problem.

My wife and I both attended the family workshop weekend at the end of camp. I will say that it should be mandatory because the parents have just as much to do with the success with the program as the child does. It was very eye opening. I did get the opportunity to sit down at lunch and dinner with the president/co-founder of Wellspring (you!) and was able to ask a lot of questions. I appreciated your time and insight.

I had concerns about why Steve would eat so much and was worried that he might be depressed or have some other emotional issue. His Behavioral Coach told me that Steve was very well adjusted and ate because he just wanted food due to his powerful biology more than anything else. That means that his weight problem had more to do with what we fed him—and his genes/ biological tendency to gain weight easily.

The ride home from camp was tough. We were not prepared very well for the trip. The snacks we had for the ride were not on plan. So it was basically Subway sandwiches and apples. When we finally got home, we had to empty all of our cupboards and the fridge. We stocked up on non-fat and extremely low-fat products. It takes time to re-write your menu. We tried just about everything to see what we liked best. You had a slogan at the training that was something like this "find lovable foods that love you back." That is basically what we have lived by since coming home from camp.

The day after we got home, Steve had a team baseball party at our house. This was very important to him. He was torn because Wellspring made an offer to extend his stay two more weeks and he had such a great time and made some great friends. However, he gave up being on the all-star team in baseball to go to Wellspring and this party meant a lot to him. We took the advice from Wellspring that "kids will eat healthy if that is what is presented to them." We had melon, watermelon, fat-free brownies, fat-free rice crispy treats, fat-free hot dogs, salad with fat-free dressing for the team party on the day after we returned from camp. This was another big boost for Steve. His friends and coaches were amazed at the transformation and the food was all eaten with no complaints; so, Steve did not have to feel like he was different.

We found a local Bison farm and we buy bison burger for hamburgers, which is even leaner than lean beef. We always have fresh fruit, yogurt, Jello and other "free foods" around to eat. There has not been a high-fat cookie, cake, or anything of that sort in our house for three and a half years. Any desserts we have are homemade cakes or treats that have zero or near-zero fat. Unfortunately, I have a sweet tooth, but I will not bring any junk into the house for Steve's sake.

Obviously, we have the issue with Steve visiting friends and spending the night. We would go over the plan with his friends' parents and sometimes send food with Steve that he could eat just to be sure he is not hungry. We have some very good friends that really supported him and accommodated him while he would visit. Most people know at this point that he only eats healthy, very low-fat foods. Our friends and family make mistakes sometimes, but they mean well. I try to explain it like this to people: imagine you had Celiac disease and you could not eat gluten. Those people have to change their diet or die. We treat fat for Steve like gluten. We have to eliminate it. He cannot eat it. It is his gluten. I hope that makes sense.

Obviously, there is some fat in the diet. Even vegetarians must find it hard to avoid it at some level. And the word Moderation is not in our vocabulary. Moderation doesn't work. It takes a healthy obsession to beat this problem. That is something that many people do not understand.

At this point, we really don't do much for Steve. Our shopping habits have been modified; we know what to buy; we know what is good to eat. So, it is pretty easy. My wife and I also eat the same way as Steve and both of us have lost a lot of weight. We are not as good as Steve because he has a mental log of everything he eats and really does not crave junk food. He is amazing! He likes low-fat smoothies; he loves fruit. He has changed. It is a big commitment. Healthy food costs more; fresh fruit and veggies can add up, but we and Steve know what the alternative is. So, we all want to do what is right for his heath, and ours.

I think in general, friends and family understand his struggle. They will ask us what they should make, what can he have? You cannot run away from it, you have to say, I am sorry, I cannot eat that. Then you can ask, Do you have something else I might have?

We do not eat out much anymore unless we are traveling. Lunch is usually Jimmy Johns or Subway and for dinner, we try to find a BD's Mongolian BBQ. BD's is awesome for Steve. Everything is healthy. You can build your dinner online and get the calories and fat before you make your meal, but most of it is veggies, so it is all free food so he can eat well and not be hungry. We also will review menus online for local restaurants where we will be visiting and make our decisions on where to eat based on the healthiness of the menu. We also have found a local Pizzeria that has fat-free cheese. That is a life saver, because every once in a while, you gotta have pizza. In fact, if we have guests, we won't even tell them it is fat free and no one knows the difference.

We also have Mongolian BBQ night at home; we cut up all different veggies, shrimp, chicken, squash, onions, you name it, then everyone fills their bowl with veggies and shimp and chicken. We have a large griddle; you pick your favorite seasoning, soy sauce or teriyaki, salt, pepper, garlic, all fat free, and then throw it on the griddle just like at the restaurant. It is a huge hit. Steve's hockey team loves it.

Those are some of the things we have done. Parents just have to change, too.

I am doing this because I think you have a wonderful program and your people are great. You saved Steve's life. What more can I say. Sorry if my thoughts are a little scattered, but it's an emotional thing to write about and I am very passionate about it. Thanks again for all you have done.

Sincerely,
Dave M

Steve's Perspective 2018: Five Keys to My Success

1. **OBEDIENCE:** Sticking to my diet and workout regimens.
2. **HARD WORK:** Pushing myself harder every day.
3. **PREPARATION:** Preparing meals and workout plans helps me reach my personal goals.
4. **DEDICATION:** Making sure I dedicate time every day to my workouts and eating plan.
5. **FOCUS:** Setting new short-term goals and staying focused on accomplishing those goals.

TRICIA H.

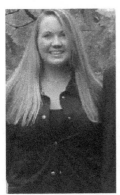

BEFORE:
2006: 194 lbs.
2018: 127 lbs.

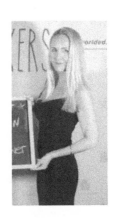

2013 Perspective

Growing up, I was a normal-sized girl with a little bit of a tummy. Throughout elementary and middle school, I was somewhat active and played soccer, tennis, and golf. But things changed when I turned sixteen and I started boarding school, and that is when I began to gain weight. I was not as active as I had been in middle school and I had access to a variety of fattening foods both on and off campus. I ate when I was bored or sad.

By the end of my sophomore year, my parents were concerned about my weight. My mother approached me with the idea of attending Wellspring New York, an all-girls fitness/weight-loss camp that summer. I liked the idea and began my first summer in 2006 (when I was sixteen years old) at Wellspring New York for the full eight weeks.

My life changed that summer. I found a passion for fitness classes, jogging, and a community that supported and encouraged my weight-loss. I learned to manage the foods I loved and shift them into healthier very low-fat versions, which further contributed to my weight loss. That first summer, I lost twenty pounds, reshaped my body and my mind set through exercise and classes, and transformed my life. While I had gotten my weight down from 194 to 174, I still had more to lose in order to be a healthy weight for my age, size, and frame. I continued jogging when I got back to school and made running a part of my daily routine. I lost another ten pounds my junior year at school, and the summer before my senior year I decided to return to Wellspring to get off the last ten to fifteen pounds I wanted to lose. Starting my senior year, I was down to 150 and felt great. I have maintained a weight between 140 and 150 for the last six years and that has transformed my life.

2018 Perspective: Thinking My Way Thin

Healthy Obsession

My healthy obsession has been learning to take care of myself—mind and body. That includes being kind to myself and finding ways to manage stress that don't include eating. This has meant music on the elliptical, shopping at local farmers' markets, reading, hip-hop classes, and meditation via an app. I'm happier and healthier when I say "yes" to me and "no" sometimes to others. That's just part of being a weight controller. I've learned to worry less about what others think—about my food choices or if I say no to last-minute after work happy hours. I love being social, but I also love to feel good; prioritizing my health and well-being has helped me succeed mentally and physically in my weight loss journey, which is invaluable.

Five Keys to My Success

1. **LOVING TO MOVE:** Avoid getting stuck with something that you don't enjoy. This makes movement a surprisingly fun process and increases confidence along the way.

2. **MOTIVATION IS THE BEST DIET:** When I decided to lose weight, that moment changed my life. I realized I never wanted for feel unhappy with my weight again. Sometimes this requires

uncovering the reasons you avoid exercise or perhaps eat unhealthy food in solitude. Joining a group or even having someone to talk to can be pretty helpful, too.

3. **FOOD MONITORING:** Self-monitoring everything you put in your mouth—even if it's something you're not proud of—will keep you accountable to yourself. It helps you identify trends in your eating patterns, food, stressors, weight, and areas of improvement.

4. **PLAN AHEAD:** Planning helps with your schedule, diet, social events, holidays, drinking, and travel. This helps with finding healthy foods that you love, like turkey jerky and sugar-free mocha in my coffee.

5. **STAY POSITIVE AND REALISTIC:** It's not a sprint; it's a marathon. I had zero expectations for the first summer I attended a weight-loss camp. However, with renowned clinical psychologist Dr. Kirschenbaum as one our camp's founders—I trusted the program. I've lost sixty-seven pounds and kept it off for twelve years. Based on my weight-loss journey, I can honestly say that if you're patient, work hard, and hold yourself accountable—then results will come.

SERGEANT TONY

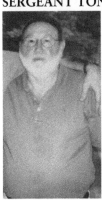

Weight loss of 55 lbs.—maintained for 3 years (as of 2018)

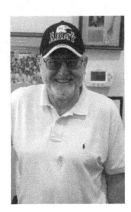

Tony was a combat veteran in Vietnam who was seriously wounded. He recovered to become a successful manager in a large company, form a close supportive relationship with his wife of many years, raise a healthy and happy family, and become a remarkably dedicated organizer of veteran-related reunions and group meetings.

Healthy Obsession

My healthy obsession means that I'm very consistently focused, every day, and I do not feel deprived with the type of food I eat (very low fat).

Seven Keys to Success

1. **HARD WORK:** Willingness to work hard at this It's not easy or magical, but it can be done.
2. **DISCIPLINED:** Smart hard work, and for me, knowing that it's okay not to eat lunch most of the time.
3. **EDUCATION:** About key goals (very low fat, step goals, self-monitoring).
4. **SELF-MONITORING 100%:** to see variations that impact weight and learn how to interpret what I eat.
5. **GREAT SUPPORT AT HOME:** My wife has been a creative, eager partner, looking at labels carefully and cooking great creative very low-fat foods.
6. **CONSISTENCY OF EATING AND EXERCISING:** focusing every day on the plan/goals.
7. **THE RIGHT TOOLS:** professional consultation and reading, learning from Dr. Kirschenbaum how to master this very challenging aspect of living.

CHAPTER 2
Nature and Nurture of the Seven Stymie Beasts

et's consider now how cognitive biases help create and maintain all seven Stymie Beasts. That first involves listing and explaining the nature of the ten types of cognitive biases, with their implications for weight controllers. Then, I will present each of the seven Stymie Beasts and identify the specific cognitive biases that helped create and sustain them.

TEN COGNITIVE BIASES	
Affect	Making choices based on **feelings** more than analysis: "The emotional tail wags the rational dog".
Anchoring	**First** piece of information becomes more important than anything else.
Availability	**WYSIATI**—What You See Is All There Is: Gives great power to commercials, dominant ideas or programs readily available.
Confirmation	Seeking and attending primarily/only to information that **conforms** with our existing way of thinking about something.
Conservation	Favoring **current** approaches despite new evidence favoring new or different approaches; resistence to shifting paradigms.

Innovation	The opposite of conservatism: Favoring something just because it's **new,** not because the evidence suggests it's better than current approaches.
Outcome	Basing decisions on **outcomes** regardless of how the outcome was achieved (luck > science, logic).
Overconfidence	Over-valuing our impulses or instinctive beliefs or **guesses;** expecting our ideas to work out right regardless of the actual challenges we face; viewing our ideas through very rose-colored glasses.
Recency	Focusing on and remembering the **latest** information, what was heard or experienced more recently, more than information or experiences from earlier times.
Representative	Greatly exaggerating the commonness of something just based on **experiencing** it or seeing it, rather than rely on base rate statistics or systematic analysis of the quality of information.

TABLE 2-1

Affect

DEFINITION: Making decisions based on feelings primarily and not based on systematic analysis or facts.

Dr. Daniel Kahneman described the affect bias by noting that such a bias happens when the answer to an easy question ("How do I feel about it?") provides the answer to a much harder question ("What do I think about it?"). Psychologist Paul Slovic and colleagues demonstrated this bias by providing information to people about various technologies. For example, the researchers wrote a paragraph about fluoridation of water and preservatives in foods. When participants read about the numerous benefits of such technologies, they changed their views of the risks of such technologies—after first rating them high in risk, they changed to rating them as low in risk. These changed views of risks and benefits seemed especially noteworthy to Dr. Kahneman because the participants made changes in their views despite receiving no new information upon which to make those changes. They simply liked the technologies more after reading those paragraphs and then decided they liked everything about them. That liking preference produced decision making biased by feeling more favorably about something—an affective bias.

<u>IMPLICATIONS FOR WEIGHT CONTROL:</u> Some diets encourage people to eat things that other diets (and good sense) deter them from eating. For example, low-carb diets encourage people to eat high-fat foods like cheeseburgers as long as they bypass the buns. That can produce a certain euphoria in long-term dieters. Other approaches often make it sound like weight controllers can implement their plans with much less effort than it usually takes to succeed. For example, one well-known advertisement says:

"Never any weighing, measuring,
or counting calories or points."

The positive affect (excitement) created by these prospects can sway weight controllers to try their methods, despite the ton of science that strongly argues against their utility.

ANCHORING

<u>DEFINITION:</u> Making decisions based on the first piece of information that becomes known to the decision maker—information that may help (or may not help) solve a problem.

Anchoring has undoubtedly helped some poorly qualified applicants get hired for jobs. The first person who seems plausible for some jobs, gets the okay before employers fully consider other options. In a similar vein, the first solution proposed to solve problems gets undue attention in various settings.

<u>IMPLICATIONS FOR WEIGHT CONTROL:</u> If a weight controller decides to lose weight, then the first approach that comes to mind or that he or she sees may become the one to use. People talk about Atkins-style low-carb/high-fat diets quite often. The science doesn't support

the value of that approach (as we will review in subsequent chapters), but if that exposure becomes an anchor, then the weight controller may well go for it. That's unfortunate, but part of a very common method of solving problems—in this case, one that can fuel Stymie Beasts.

Availability

DEFINITION: Readily available information can lead to misinformation and decisions affected by such inaccurate perceptions.

We are exposed to information based on its appeal, its distinctiveness, its familiarity and availability, and, quite often, by the capability of the owners of products to pay for frequent and compelling commercials. Drs. Khaneman and Tversky and their colleagues used an acronym to summarize part of this process: What You See Is All There Is (WYSIATI). That's the information that's most *available* to us, and such availability influences our perceptions and decisions in powerful ways.

Psychologists Paul Slovic, Sarah Lichtenstein, and Baruch Fischhoff conducted important studies on the availability bias. Consider your answers to the questions about death that they asked many people. Then, read Table 2-2 to see what the participants believed versus the realities of recent data:

- **Strokes:** Do accidents cause more deaths than strokes?
- **Tornadoes:** Do tornadoes cause more deaths than asthma?
- **Diseases:** Do diseases cause more deaths than accidents?

| CAUSES OF DEATH: BELIEFS VS. REALITY ||
BELIEFS	**REALITY**
• Strokes less likely to kill than accidents	• Strokes TWICE as likely to kill than accidents
• Tornadoes more likely to kill than asthma	• Asthma kills 20 times more often than tornadoes
• Disease kills about as often as accidents	• Disease kills 18 times more often than accidents

TABLE 2-2

IMPLICATIONS FOR WEIGHT CONTROL: In the case of the beliefs in Table 2-2, most people see more accidents on television than they see victims of strokes. They also see and hear about tornadoes on television more often than asthma. That makes most of us think that accidents and tornadoes kill far more often than diseases like strokes and asthma. Mistaken beliefs like these can seriously affect decisions we make, including decisions about how to lose weight.

Here's another more colloquial way of thinking about the availability bias: "Them that has, gets." That bird in the hand is worth two in the bush. Those ideas and products that are right in front of us get most of the attention. For example, low-carb diets get advertised every day—and have been getting tremendous amounts of attention in the media in recent years. Yet no major health organization ever recommended low-carb diets, because the scientific evidence does not support the benefits of such an approach. Yet most people seem to believe such an approach works far better than the much more consistently endorsed method—low-fat or very low-fat diets.

CONFIRMATION

DEFINITION: Seeking out, focusing on, and remembering information that confirms what we already believe.

In 1962, Dr. Thomas Kuhn, an iconic physicist and philosopher, published one of the most important books about science ever written: *The Structure of Scientific Revolutions*. That book taught us a lot about how people, including scientists, resist new ways of thinking about things. As an example of that, he reviewed the findings of a study that he noted "deserves to be far better known outside of the trade [meaning by psychologists]" (p.62).

In 1949, psychologists J.S. Bruner and Leo Postman published a study that shows a great example of confirmation bias. Dr. Kuhn put it this way: "Novelty emerges only with difficulty, manifested by resistance ..." (p.64). This means that accepting new and different ideas/beliefs creates a certain amount of anxiety in many of us. Our worlds seem more unstable and unpredictable when new ideas make themselves known, perhaps after considerable resistance.

The Bruner and Postman study helped make that point remarkably well. These researchers created a deck of cards that included many normal cards, but also a number of cards that did not conform to usual expectations. For example, they created a red six of spades (instead of the usual black one) and a black four of hearts (instead of a red one). Dr. Kuhn called these the "anomalous" cards. Experimenters gave the subjects a card, took the card away, and then asked for the identification of that card. Then experimenters did that with two cards, then three, and so on until subjects were receiving several cards in a row to identify.

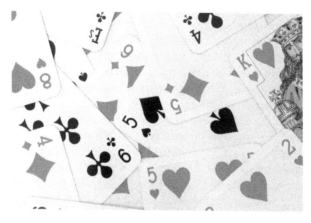

Subjects identified the normal cards correctly but ignored the strange qualities of the anomalous cards. They seemed completely unaware of the strangeness of those cards and identified them as if they were all perfectly normal. So, instead of saying that the red six of spades was red, they just called it a six of spades. After many repeated exposures to those anomalous cards, most subjects started calling them out with some hesitation. For example, they might say that the red six of spades had something wrong with it—a red border. Finally, most started getting the identifications of the strange cards correct. A few subjects, however, were never able to make the requisite adjustment to identify the anomalous cards accurately. As Dr. Kuhn explained it, "Even at forty times, the average exposure required to recognize the abnormal cards ..., more than ten percent of the anomalous cards were not correctly identified."

Confirmation bias quite simply distorted the participants' perception of the cards. In many cases, they simply *did not* recognize the change in images despite many exposures to them. Something within them caused them to confirm their expectations of the colors of those strange cards, ignoring the evidence of their own eyes.

Here's another great example of confirmation bias: https://www.quora.com/What-are-some-good-examples-of-a-confirmation-bias. In this example, a reporter tells interviewees that he has a rule that applies to the following numbers: 2, 4, 8. What do you think the next three numbers that fit the rule might be? What is the rule?

Most people believe the rule is this: keep multiplying each of the numbers by two: start with the 2, then 2 X 2 = 4, then 4 X 2 = 8. Interviewees would then offer a bunch of numbers in sequence that match that multiply by two rule, e.g., 16, 32, 64 (8 X 2, then 16 X 2, and finally, 32 X 2). The reporter in the video mentioned above kept telling the participants that these numbers did indeed follow the rule he had in mind. However, the rule wasn't to keep multiplying the numbers by two.

So, what was the rule?

The answer: List three numbers, any three numbers, in ascending order. The confirmation bias shows up by people continuing to suggest a sequence of numbers that fit the "multiply by two" rule. They didn't try other rules, but just kept asking about three numbers that fit their belief about the rule—over and over again. Some just could not figure out the simple answer at all!

Here's the essence of confirmation bias: *We often see only what we want or expect to see.*

IMPLICATIONS FOR WEIGHT CONTROL: Most people have strong beliefs about what works for weight control. They develop these beliefs over time by experimenting themselves, watching commercials, reading, and ostensibly learning from the experience of others. The fifty- to one-hundred-billion-dollar diet industry keeps making powerful commercials, supports certain research studies, and tries to get into people's heads about this—with considerable success. Then, the search for confirming evidence takes over: Keep reinforcing what you think you know about how to do this. That decreases the openness to new or better ideas, unfortunately. This thinking leads many people to think white potatoes and bread are the enemies because they don't fit within a low-carb or low-glycemic index diet. Actually, they're both very low in fat and can work well for weight controllers.

CONSERVATISM

<u>DEFINITION:</u> Favoring existing approaches despite compelling evidence that supports making changes.

Similar in many ways to confirmation bias, conservatism bias resists new, and in this case, better ideas. Confirmation bias specifically favors one's own existing beliefs, seeking confirmation of those beliefs. Conservatism bias more generally resists change regardless of one's own beliefs. For example, you can get used to living in a very cramped home in an unpleasant and even dangerous neighborhood. Even though you have enough money to make an upward move, your conservatism bias keeps you firmly in place. Uncomfortable and risky though it might be, that's where you might choose to stay.

<u>IMPLICATIONS FOR WEIGHT CONTROL:</u> As of this writing, low-carb diets have dominated the dietary airways for about twenty years. Scientists and other experts consistently argue against pursuit of this approach, but many people resist the argument against low-carb diets because of conservatism bias. Perhaps some of this perspective borrows from a famous saying, "The enemy you know is always better than the enemy you don't know."

INNOVATION

<u>DEFINITION:</u> The opposite of conservatism bias: Favoring new or innovative ideas, regardless of the science or logic behind them.

Advertisers for almost every product seem fully aware of the innovation bias. How many times have you seen the exact same food or detergent wrapped in a different box or color scheme with the word "New" blazing at you, just begging you to go for it again, hoping to ignite your enthusiasm for the new wine in old bottles. In the golf industry, every single year, companies promote their supposedly new innovations to promote sales of revised equipment. This annual ritual results in golfers spending millions on new drivers and new golf balls hoping to get a few extra yards of distance by using the ostensible latest and greatest. Objective tests would show them, however, that the shiny new clubs and balls rarely produce major improvements to their games.

Unfortunately, innovations can prove worse than their predecessors in some cases. For example, when laparoscopic surgery first became available, many surgeries using the smaller incisions facilitated by impressive new cameras produced notably worse outcomes for thousands of people than the prior "open surgery" approaches, particularly when laparoscopic procedures first gained favor. For example, even a relatively recent paper by Dr. V. Velanovich, published in *Surgical Endoscopy* in 2000, reported worse outcomes for laparoscopic hernia repairs compared to open surgery.

Implications for Weight Control: Arguments against low-fat diets illustrate the unfortunate consequences of innovation bias for weight controllers. A great many diet gurus and even scientists made the anti-low-fat argument by citing the focus on low-fat diets in the 1980s. They asserted that the tremendous enthusiasm for such diets as the *T-Factor Diet* (published in 1989) caused an increase in degree of obesity in this country in the subsequent decades. The argument goes something like this: "We tried that approach and look what happened! The obesity epidemic accelerated!"

This argument comes from what's called, in statistics, a spurious correlation. Indeed, obesity did increase following a wave of enthusiasm for low-fat diets. However, the population did not actually change its eating habits despite the expressed enthusiasm in books and articles for low-fat eating. In the US, people continued to eat an average of eighty fat grams per day in the 1980s through to the present day. They did not lower fat intake to the recommended levels in these low-fat/very low-fat diets (generally less than thirty grams of fat per day for most people). Many other factors contributed to the accelerating obesity epidemic over those decades, like increasingly sedentary living (e.g., the invention of the internet, laptops, smart phones) and the continuing availability of inexpensive high-fat foods advertised aggressively as part of the good life.

Just because new supposed solutions argue vehemently against very low-fat diets, does that mean that such low-fat diets don't work anymore? Nope!

OUTCOME

<u>DEFINITION</u>: Basing decisions on outcomes regardless of the process used to produce the outcomes.

Gambling produces winners quite often. Every state lottery yields positive outcomes occasionally. Those who buy the omnipresent state lottery tickets get very excited when they win. Somehow, they manage to forget *how* they won the occasional ten or twenty dollars. They won by investing many times more than those winnings on losing tickets. Ask any lottery player about their winnings/losings and you will hear echoes of this exact story. The players will recount their glorious victorious moments but have difficulty remembering the dozens or hundreds of disappointing days that preceded the small victories. The term "Gambler's Fallacy" reflects this pattern: keep investing in bets and you're bound to win some—but you lose a lot more than you win overall.

IMPLICATIONS FOR WEIGHT CONTROL: You *can* lose weight for sure doing any one of the following things:
- Fast for several days.
- Eat only low-fat hot dogs for a week (maximum of ten per day)
- Walk/run thirty minutes a day, every day, and keep your calories under 1,000 per day.
- Eat only low-fat protein shakes (total of less than 1,000 calories per day).

Just because each of these unreasonable and unsustainable approaches *can* produce weight loss:
1. Does that justify using any of them?
2. What happens to your overall health by eating in the ways suggested here, for example?
3. Can you really sustain these approaches for days, weeks, months, and years?

In a beautifully elegant way, science can answer all of these questions. The answers to the three questions posed above are:
1. No;
2. Nothing good; and
3. No. Understanding the science of weight control can provide a pathway to lifelong weight control (final five chapters). Focusing only on a friend's supposed way to produce favorable outcomes (without scientific evidence of its efficacy) will put you on a path to failure in the vast majority of cases.

OVERCONFIDENCE

DEFINITION: Unrealistically positive views of one's own knowledge, skills, and judgment can lead to mistakes in decision making.

Psychologist Shelly Taylor and her associates demonstrated that most people use positive biases (what they termed "positive illusions") when evaluating themselves. These positive illusions include unrealistic optimism, exaggerated perceptions of their own control/ mastery of various tasks, and generally overly positive self-evaluations. In contrast, depressed people often seem "sadder, but wiser." They judge themselves more realistically than well-adjusted people. That realistic judgment reveals flaws in performance that contribute to a sadder, more pessimistic outlook. Positive illusions (even positive delusions) may improve adjustment to life's challenges by making the world seem more favorable, predictable, and encouraging. These tendencies may indeed improve adjustment, but such biases can lead to all sorts of mistakes in decision making.

For example, my colleagues, Drs. DeDe Owens and Ed O'Connor, and I looked at choices made by golfers when selecting which club to hit for a couple of tee shots. Based on recommendations from expert golfers/instructors, the tee shots studied would produce much better outcomes if golfers chose clubs that hit the ball shorter distances. In other words, shorter clubs with more loft are much easier to control. What we found seemed amazing. *Ten times as many golfers chose longer hitting clubs versus their shorter hitting clubs!* When given the recommendation to use the shorter clubs, big surprise: the shots turned out significantly better. Almost all of these golfers, a large sample of amateur players (385 of them), simply used positive illusions that had them convinced that they could go for much more difficult, longer shots and do just fine. Oops—scores go up when golfers make such mistakes.

IMPLICATIONS FOR WEIGHT CONTROL: Overconfidence can also lead people to think they know more than they really do about a host of things, including choices about how best to lose weight. This time the "oops" created by such cognitive biases can produce unfortunate consequences for their health and well-being. Sometimes we don't know what we don't know.

Recency

DEFINITION: Making choices based on most recent experiences, regardless of the importance of prior experiences. In other words, we favor recency in our decision making more than a systematic analysis would suggest.

Featured Research: Choosing More, Not Less, Pain Sometimes

Pursuing weight loss requires a choice: Deciding to make changes in your life to pursue a challenging goal. This book focuses on how to get yourself to elect to take on that challenge, despite the demands it makes on you.

Researchers have studied such choices and sometimes found surprising factors that influence our decision making. For example, psychologists Daniel Kahneman, Barbara Frederickson, and Charles Schreiber, and physician Donald Redelmeier had participants place their hands in painfully cold, but tolerable, water, one hand at a time. This cold-hand situation lasted 60 seconds at 57°F for one hand (followed by a warm towel) or 90 seconds, 57°F for 60 seconds and then 55°F for the last 30 seconds for the other hand. Experimenters told participants that after those first two trials of the cold-hand task, they would get a third trial. Participants then chose which type of trial they wanted for the third trial: the 60-second or 90-second versions. They all realized that the 90-second version was longer, but 80% of those who noticed a warming feeling for the last 30 seconds of the 90-second version opted to repeat that one instead of much shorter 60-second trial (as shown below).

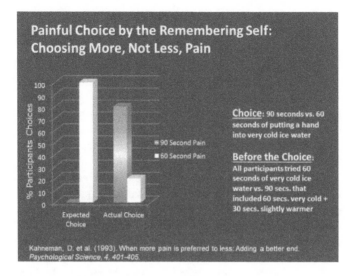

Painful Choice by the Remembering Self: Choosing More, Not Less, Pain

Choice: 90 seconds vs. 60 seconds of putting a hand into very cold ice water

Before the Choice: All participants tried 60 seconds of very cold ice water vs. 90 secs. that included 60 secs. very cold + 30 secs. slightly warmer

Kahneman, D. et al. (1993). When more pain is preferred to less: Adding a better end. Psychological Science, 4, 401–405.

Doesn't it seem that if you participated in this study, you would select the shorter duration of pain (60 seconds instead of 90 seconds)? Most chose the longer trial because they apparently remembered (and accentuated in their memories) the more comfortable warming up period at the end of their 90-second trial. These participants followed certain principles that can apparently impact our decision making. The authors called those principles "peak-end rule" and "duration neglect." It seems that quite often we tend to ignore the duration of unpleasant experiences and focus more on the more recent aspects of them when remembering them.

IMPLICATIONS FOR WEIGHT CONTROL: Recent experiences can deter enthusiasm for sustained efforts toward change. If a weight controller fails at an approach, that failure can lead to hopelessness about the possibility of finding a better approach. Such recent experiences can blind weight controllers to the possibility of success.

REPRESENTATIVE

DEFINITION: Ignoring or minimizing base rate information when making predictions about outcomes.

Many decisions involve making guesses about the chances of something happening. When watching sporting events, you might try to guess who will win—might even bet on that. To win most bets like that, it helps to know the base rates. A base rate is the usual outcome associated with a team or individual. Betting parlors give much lower odds for those who win a great deal, for example.

What about buying a car? Some car buyers study *Consumer Reports* to determine if the car they find appealing seems generally reliable. If you make reliability a big deal in such purchases, you would tend to buy cars with histories of staying functional and minimizing repairs over time: Toyotas and Hondas vs. Mercedes and Chryslers, for example.

Dr. Daniel Kahneman and his research partner, the late Dr. Amos Tversky, defined representative bias as ignoring or minimizing base rate information when making decisions. Many stereotypical ways of thinking get that way due to base rates that emerge in certain directions. For example, very tall and thin athletes play more basketball than very short agile/flexible people, the latter of whom might turn to gymnastics much more often than basketball. Another stereotype that works: Young men drive much more aggressively than elderly women, most of the time.

So, what happens when you make decisions regardless of base rate information (representativeness)? You usually lose—but not always!

Bowling Example

A group of my friends and I bowl quite often together, just for fun (and for modest $2 side bets) and in league competitions. The photo below shows a group of us that won our twenty-four-week league championship in 2016, quite an exciting occasion:

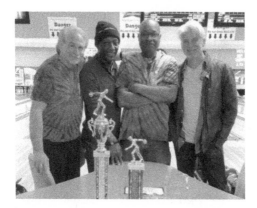

I'm the guy on your left (hand on a chair) as you view this and the person in this example, my friend named Keith, stands on the right (hands in pockets).

One day Keith faced a very difficult split. Bowling involves ten frames in which bowlers can knock down all pins on their first shot (getting a strike, the best one can do) or get a second shot to knock down any remaining pins (to get a spare, the second best you can do). Keith had a split for his second shot (pins numbered nine and ten); a split is a grouping of pins that has at least a one pin gap between the pins. Keith had knocked down the eight other pins with his first ball. The image below shows a ball hitting the number three pin head on. Just to the right of the three pin and behind it (in the back row) is the nine pin. The pin in the right corner of the image is the ten pin. With only the nine and ten pins on the lane, you can see that a pretty big gap exists between those pins—making the required shot to get a spare (worth a bonus of ten pins) quite difficult.

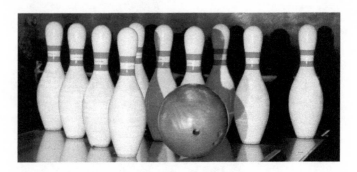

Keith averages about 138, meaning he's a pretty good bowler but not a great one. My educated guess was that the base rate for Keith to convert this split was about ten to one against him knocking down both pins in one shot (i.e., making the spare). So, I offered Keith a bet, giving him five-to-one odds against his making this shot ($10 to be paid to him by me if he made it; $2 to be paid by him to me if he did not). Well, sorry to say, Keith defied the base rate odds, which certainly can happen; he converted that very tough split and jubilantly pocketed $10 of my money.

Two weeks later, another unusual thing happened during bowling. Keith beat me during a league competition in one game: 154 to 151. I average 177 to Keith's 138. In the approximately 150 times that we've bowled together, Keith probably scored better than me two games in a row only three or four times. That made the odds for Keith to beat me in the next game about twenty to one against. This time, I offered Keith a three-to-one bet ($6 from me to him if he wins, $2 from him to me if he loses), banking on the representative bias. That is, because Keith just won a game, it seemed quite possible that he would ignore the base rate data and greatly overestimate his odds of winning a second game in a row. Even though Keith is a very smart man and great with numbers (an experienced accountant), I was hoping representative bias would kick in—helping me earn some revenge for the money lost when Keith made that amazing split.

Sure enough, Keith took the bet, accepted the unreasonably low three-to-one odds without even arguing for five-to-one or higher. Guess what happened? This time the representative base rate proved itself to be what it usually is: a good predictor of outcomes (i.e., representative of the likely outcome). Keith bowled a 132 versus my 190, netting me a tiny bit of revenge ($2 of the $10 lost on the previous bet that Keith won by making the nine-ten split). Surprisingly, at least to me, a similar scenario emerged a couple of weeks after Keith lost this bet. He once again out-bowled me in a game. When offered the same three-to-one odds for the next game (three-to-one against the possibility of out-bowling me in the subsequent game), he took the bet again. Same outcome: Keith lost this bet again—and again by a substantial margin.

<u>IMPLICATIONS FOR WEIGHT CONTROL</u>: Someone's success with a particular diet may predict very little of what that diet can probably do for you. The low-carb diet craze has netted many millions of dollars for its champions because of this factor. People lose weight quickly when they virtually eliminate carbohydrates from their diets. How? It takes a fair amount of liquid to digest carbohydrates. Loss of such liquid upon initiating this unfortunate diet can cause a three- to five-pound weight loss in a day or two. Friends and neighbors start talking to each other excitedly about this "amazing weight loss" and, lo and behold, people start gravitating toward it. Then, when they look sideways at a bagel, the weight starts piling back on and stays there. Low-carb fans pursue this approach by ignoring the failures and over-emphasizing the short-term weight losses. They do this despite the scientific evidence and consensus by virtually every expert group that low-carb diets generally do not work and usually prove more harmful than helpful.

SEVEN STYMIE BEASTS

CAN'T

"I CAN'T LOSE WEIGHT. I'VE TRIED EVERYTHING; I'M JUST TIRED OF THE ROLLER COASTER—LOSE WEIGHT, FEEL GREAT, GAIN IT ALL BACK AND THEN SOME, AND FEEL LIKE CRAP. I'VE TRIED EVERY DIET AND PROGRAM; NOTHING WORKS FOR ME. I'M DONE."

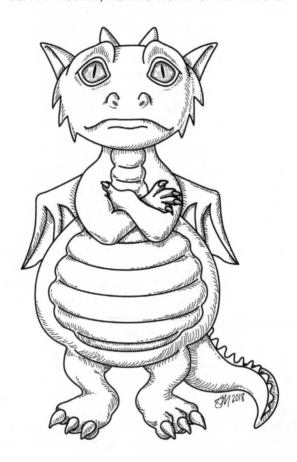

<u>COGNITIVE BIASES:</u> Availability, Conservatism, Representative

Most widely available weight loss materials and programs simply do not base themselves on science. They exist more to make money than to help people make major changes in their lifestyles and health. The Can't Beast emerges when people fail using available approaches destined to fail, like low-carb diets or whole food approaches without any support (availability bias). Conservation bias kicks in because people often choose methods with which they've become familiar, something they grew up hearing about or have seen others use in the past. These weight controllers don't usually search for scientific evidence to document the success/failure base rates for these approaches. They just go for it. A systemic search for data would show far more failures than successes with these conservative and widely available approaches. Ignoring the data (representative bias) allows for trying, once again, an approach destined to fail.

ADDICT

"I HAVE TO HAVE MY CHOCOLATE FIX EVERY DAY; I JUST HAVE TO. PEANUT BUTTER ALSO CALLS OUT TO ME EVERY DAY. I'VE TRIED LOSING WEIGHT AND KNOW THAT WOULD BE A GOOD THING. I JUST CAN'T GET PAST MY ADDICTION TO THESE CERTAIN FOODS. I'VE COME TO JUST ACCEPT THAT AS PART OF MY REALITY."

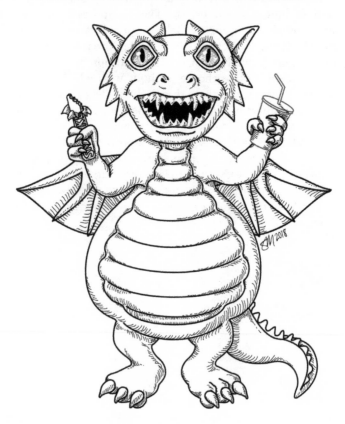

<u>**COGNITIVE BIASES:**</u> Affect, Confirmation, Outcome

Emotion dominates this Addict Stymie Beast (affect bias). Feeling absolutely compelled to eat certain problematic foods usually involves compulsively and forcefully seeking out those foods, despite their self-destructive nature and the objections of loved ones. Then, feeling especially relieved upon eating that chocolate bar or pizza reinforces these habits—confirming their vital nature (confirmation bias) and providing the desired outcome, relief from stress (outcome bias). To change would require challenging the affect, confirmation, and outcome biases—all at once.

HATE

"There's nothing I hate more than exercising; well, maybe dieting. I just hate that feeling of pushing myself to move, sweating, getting tired, and wanting relief from all of that. I'm sort of amazed that anyone seems to like it. Maybe they're just masochists? Same thing with depriving myself of foods that I love. Where's the joy of living when you can't have beautiful tasty foods every day? It's just not for me. I agree with Mark Twain, 'Whenever I get the urge to exercise, I lie down until the feeling passes away'."

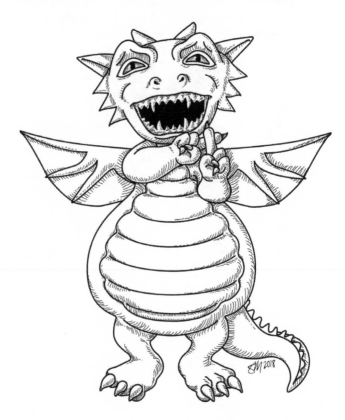

<u>COGNITIVE BIASES:</u> Affect, Recency

Certainly, invoking the word "hate" generally stirs up considerable emotion. Compare, for example, how the following two sentences make you feel:
1. I hate my younger brother!
2. I dislike my younger brother.

For most of us, the first statement seems quite ugly and inflammatory. The second just seems very common. After all, we don't get to pick our relatives. Weight controllers who espouse hatred for exercise and diet-type foods often invoke the affect bias. How can they justify something that stirs them up in such a negative way? Therefore, the affect bias can stake a strong claim to creating this Hate Stymie Beast.

Recency bias can also play a role when the weight controller struggles with exercise or eating on program. Research on long-term weight controllers shows that the process feels relatively easy six years after starting, easier than three years into it, and the latter feels quite comfortable compared to novice weight controllers. It just takes a while to get into a movement routine and find the foods on program that you really like. Recent experiences that include struggling with increasing movement or eating diet-oriented foods can bias some weight controllers against persisting in their efforts to change.

LAZY

"I KNOW IT WOULD BE REALLY GOOD FOR ME TO LOSE THIS WEIGHT, BUT I'M JUST LAZY. I JUST DON'T LIKE PUSHING MYSELF TOO HARD AND I LOVE TO SLEEP, REST, AND JUST TAKE IT EASY. I WORKED HARD IN MY LIFE AND NOW I'M JUST TIRED OF THAT. I CAN'T SEEM TO GET TOO INTERESTED IN DOING WHAT IT WOULD TAKE TO LOSE WEIGHT."

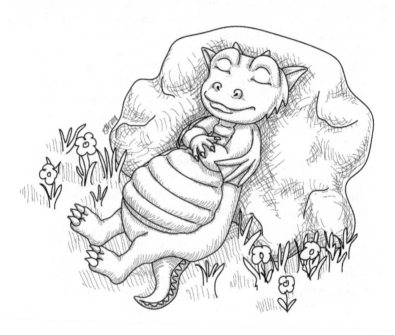

<u>COGNITIVE BIASES:</u> Affect, Recency

The Lazy Beast recalls recent efforts (recency bias) for their frustrating, annoying, unrewarding elements. This Beast nor longer focuses on how it felt to move more or achieve a difficult sub-goal, like losing a pound or two. Those feelings seemed to fade away, dominated by the negative affect (affect bias) of failures, mini-failures, and frustrations. Resisting high-fat foods, for another example, takes effort, and that feeling of deprivation can feel unpleasantly difficult.

WON'T

"LOSING WEIGHT JUST IS NOT ME. I CAN LIVE A GREAT LIFE BEING BIG—AND I STAY HEALTHY TOO. SEVERAL PEOPLE IN MY FAMILY LIVED TO BE VERY OLD DESPITE BIG WAISTLINES. SOME FAMOUS PEOPLE DID THAT TOO, LIKE ALFRED HITCHOCK AT 80, ARETHA FRANKLIN, THE QUEEN OF SOUL AT 76, AND HENRY KISSINGER, STILL WRITING POLITICAL BOOKS AT 93. BESIDES, I HAVE A RIGHT TO BE BIG. IN FACT, I'M AN ADVOCATE FOR THE CIVIL RIGHTS OF FAT PEOPLE, JUST LIKE MY FELLOW MEMBERS OF THE NATIONAL ASSOCIATION TO ADVANCE FAT ACCEPTANCE (NAAFA)."

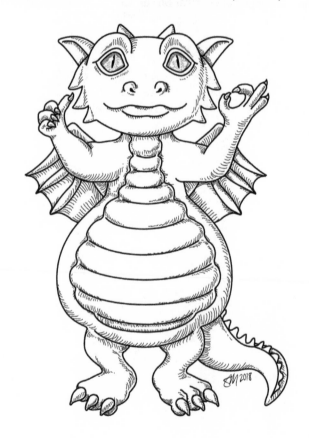

<u>COGNITIVE BIASES:</u> Representative, Confirmation, Overconfidence

NAAFA is a non-profit, all volunteer, civil rights organization founded in 1969. NAAFA is dedicated to protecting the rights and improving the quality of life for "fat people." NAAFA works to eliminate discrimination based on body size and provide "fat people" with the tools for self-empowerment through advocacy, education, and support. This is NAAFA's vision: "A society in which people of every size are accepted with dignity and equality in all aspects of life." https://www.naafaonline.com/dev2/about/

Recalling Alfred Hitchcock seems perfectly reasonable, but what about all the many obese people, famous and not so famous, who died young from complications related directly to obesity? Here are some famous examples: John Belushi, 33; John Candy, 43; Mama Cass Elliot, 34; Chris Farley, 32; and James Gandolfini, 51.

Recalling the unusual cases of very overweight people who lived long lives is a classic example of ignoring the base rates—or representative bias. Believing such an unusual outcome will happen to you if you remain overweight shows overconfidence bias—a positive prediction despite enormous odds of the negative impact on health of excess weight. Confirmation bias plays a role when joining an organization like NAAFA that searches for and publishes unusual findings that suggest lesser risks of obesity than scientific reality dictates. Also, relatedly, confirmation bias promotes focusing on the very real prejudices against overweight people that can obscure the focus on the negative health consequences of this disease (and it certainly is a disease).

WAITING

"I KNOW MY MOTIVATION WILL KICK IN AGAIN. I CAN FEEL IT. I LOST 75 POUNDS JUST THREE YEARS AGO. I WAS SO GUNG HO— NOTHING COULD GET IN MY WAY THEN. SOMETHING JUST GRABBED ME AND MOTIVATED ME FOR MONTHS AND MONTHS. I'M JUST WAITING FOR IT TO COME BACK AGAIN—AND I KNOW IT WILL."

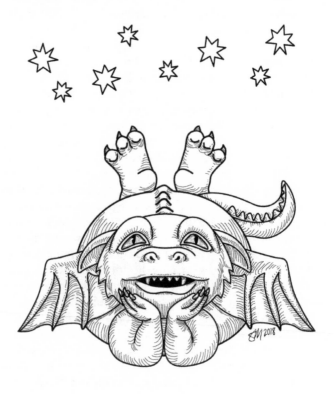

<u>COGNITIVE BIASES:</u>   Representative,   Outcome,
Availability, Conservatism, Overconfidence

Five of the ten cognitive biases seem active in creating
the Waiting Beast. That suggests how far removed from
reasonable this Beast lives and breathes. Motivation
describes the "whys" of behavior. What motivates us
to drive somewhat close to the speed limit? Dangers of
speeding and anxiety about expensive tickets that could
threaten our licenses motivates many of us when we are
behind the wheels of our cars. In places that ignore most
speed limits, like Germany's autobahn, many drivers exceed
100 mph routinely—something that rarely happens in the
US. Those autobahn drivers step on the gas with impunity
partly because avoiding tickets isn't part of their motivation.
Motivation to work hard to lose weight happens for
tangible reasons, too. Something I witnessed hundreds
of times helps to clarify this point. I had the privilege of
designing weight loss camps and boarding schools for
overweight young people (primarily teenagers), called
Wellspring. For many years, Wellspring was the leading
provider of treatment services for overweight young people
in the US. In Wellspring's programs, many young people
at first seemed ambivalent about working toward weight
loss. Yet when they arrived in an incredibly supportive
perfect environment for weight loss (i.e., delicious and
readily available very low-fat foods, activities organized by
others all day), they usually became excited and eager to
join in the process. Motivation changes based on available
contingencies, not just based on some internal sparkling
insight. So waiting for one's internal spark to shine generally
leaves Waiting Beasts in control, never losing their power
to block concerted efforts to lose weight.

You can probably see from this analysis how overconfidence bias (positive illusion about the spark emerging), representative bias (ignoring the fact that motivation changes when contingencies change, not by waiting for magical insights), and the others could play a role in nurturing these Waiting Beasts.

HOW?

"I really want to succeed, but I just don't know how to do it. I've tried lots of things and I still believe something out there will work for me. I keep trying the latest and what seems like the best ideas, but no luck yet. I'm just searching for that and I refuse to give up. I know people have succeeded in losing weight and keeping it off. Why not me, too?"

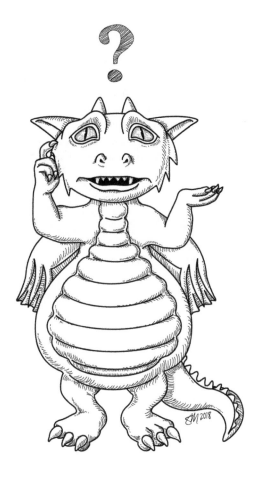

COGNITIVE BIASES: Innovation, Anchoring, Availability

Trying the latest fad diet keeps How Beasts very much alive and well. Fad diets emerge in the multi-billion-dollar diet industry not from science, but from the eagerness of their sponsors to get rich and famous. Innovation bias orients the weight controller to go for what seems new— as if new naturally makes an approach better. Science shows which approaches produce better results, not which approaches emerged most recently. New excitement from friends, neighbors, and creative marketers makes the new approaches more available (availability bias). Orienting oneself to the latest success stories enlivens anchoring bias. Those recent outcomes, or ostensible outcomes, can become dominant stories floating around in the consciousness of those wishing to find a way to succeed in this difficult quest.

CHAPTER 3
Two Ways to Tame Your Stymie Beasts

- **Therapeutic Understanding of Science (TUS)**
- **Rational Emotive Therapy (RET)**

We now know how powerful resistant forces, Stymie Beasts, emerge from biased thinking. These Beasts can pose major barriers to progress in weight control. Before presenting the five-step Very Low-Fat(VLF) Healthy Obsession Pathway (HOP) approach to losing weight most effectively (based on science, of course), let's focus on how best to tame those Stymie Beasts. We will consider two potentially powerful methods: Therapeutic Understanding of Science (TUS) and Rational Emotive Therapy (RET). After introducing both methods, we will consider how to tame each of the seven Stymie Beasts with both TUS and RET approaches.

THERAPEUTIC UNDERSTANDING OF SCIENCE (TUS)

Let's say you decided to buy a car. You saw an advertisement for a Yugo and it seemed very appealing: "Wow, such a low price [about $4,000 in 1986] for a brand new car! Probably great on gas and I bet it would stay reliable for a while—being a new car after all." You talked to a very wise, insightful friend about this decision and she said, "Hey, go with your gut." You might have even bought this car under those conditions.

Now, consider what a 1986 review of the Yugo published in the *Washington Post* reported about this same car:

> The low-priced Yugo faces a tough sell in the American market, judging from the chorus of pans it has received from automotive reviewers since it reached these shores in August.
>
> One of the severest has come from Consumer Reports magazine, which this month carried a Yugo report that read in part: "The price is the come-on for the Yugo."
>
> "Is low price sufficient for buying the Yugo?" Consumer Reports asked in its review. "We don't think so. Overall, the Yugo scored below every other small car we've tested in recent years."
>
> Motor Trend, a national auto-buff magazine, was less harsh in its criticism, but was nonetheless cool in its assessment. Of the eight new imported cars tested by the Motor Trend staff in 1986, the Yugo was ranked last, without so much as an honorable mention.

Consumer Reports provides scientifically based objective evaluations because it accepts no advertising. *Motor Trend* apparently agreed with their assessment. If you had read these types of reviews, would you buy a Yugo?

Let's take a step backward in considering this decision about the Yugo. Imagine that in 1986, the year the reviews above appeared, you decided to spend up to $7,000 on a car. Right after making that decision, you saw an advertisement for a Yugo with a bunch of excited people pictured with a new Yugo, priced at about $4,000. The anchoring bias might make that ad particularly appealing because you saw it immediately after deciding on your budget. Suddenly, that low cost might really jump out at you, begging you to consider the Yugo first and foremost. You might also just decide it seems like the right thing to do and fail to take the scientific approach to investigate base rate information about its performance and reliability (provided by *Consumer Reports*)—enacting the representative bias.

On the other hand, what if you became committed to making decisions like a scientist, especially on purchases of expensive items like cars, houses, and vacations? Two studies published in 1991 by psychologist Norbert Schwarz and his colleagues, and another one cited in that paper, showed that adopting a scientific orientation can, indeed, make people less susceptible to the influence of cognitive biases like anchoring and representative biases. Scientists analyze carefully, obtain objective data, search for base rate information, and so on. Let's get into the details next of how you can use TUS to tame those Stymie Beasts and move you closer to becoming a highly successful weight controller.

WHAT SCIENTISTS DO

Let's start this quest toward maximizing your TUS by defining science:

A group of scientists from diverse fields decided to get organized and work together to promote science: The Science Council http://sciencecouncil.org/about-us/our-definition-of-science/. They created an excellent definition of science:

*"Science is the pursuit and application
of knowledge and understanding of the
natural and social world following a systematic
methodology based on evidence."*

This definition shows both the goals of science and, most importantly, an emphasis on the method (systematic, based on evidence) of reaching those lofty goals (understanding the world). Scientists typically do the following to use that systematic methodology:

- Define things clearly, often in measurable and observable ways.
- Develop hypotheses about whatever they seek to understand based on prior scientific studies.
- Test those hypotheses using detailed descriptions of the methods used to gather data. The methods used are defined so clearly that others can repeat exactly what they did.
- Place a high value on research done using those methods, appropriate statistics, and published in peer-reviewed scientific journals. Peer-reviewed journals publish articles only after fellow scientists with expertise in the particular domain review and accept the writing, methodology, analyses, and conclusions of the paper submitted for possible publication.

Science, therefore, strives for clarity, objectivity, and thoroughness. It does not just create facts. It establishes evidence systematically that others can test for themselves. Scientists also embrace the fact that ideas, hypotheses, and seemingly clear facts can change based on new knowledge.

TRANSLATING SCIENCE INTO DECISION MAKING

If you find this approach appealing, then you would want really good sources of information to help you gather that data systematically. Steps that can help include subscribing (online or in paper) to such objective sources of information as *Consumer Reports* and *Nutrition Action Healthletter* (from the Center for Science in the Public Interest). These low-cost sources refuse to take advertising from anyone and report on a host of interesting topics related to health and well-being. They translate science for you, not perfectly or permanently, because science is dynamic. Knowledge changes as information and experiments produce new information. But these sources can give you more objective evidence about your world than you can get from Facebook postings or local news reports, and far more so than advertising.

Questions Usually Worth Asking. In addition to gathering good sources of information via certain newsletters or magazines, you can get into a habit of asking questions of the sort scientists ask routinely. These questions can apply to many decisions, like medical procedures, pills, purchases, and potential wagers with friends. The questions scientists would use when facing such decisions include:

- What are the sources of the information?
- How good are those sources of information?
- Can I see the evidence in writing?
- What are all the alternatives worth considering— and the evidence in favor or against them?

With weight management in particular, a lot of information appears every day online and in other media outlets. For example, many books become best sellers in this category, often authored by people with seemingly good credentials, like MDs. However, that's not good enough for you to decide such people meet the definition of "good sources of information."

Experts publish in peer-reviewed scientific journals. In this writer's view, a book published by anyone who does not include references to such publications within the book does not meet that expert criterion. Expert authors will always cite at least several of their own studies that have appeared in such journals. So, you can check the list of references in the book and look for the author's name. You can also look in the book or article in a website or magazine for citation of scientific studies to support the approach advocated by the supposed expert presented in such documents.

So, TUS means that you use science by gathering systematically evidence that follows from well-defined and described methods. That evidence often appears in scientific journals, and experts are those who publish in such journals, not just people with advanced degrees trying to sell you something.

RATIONAL EMOTIVE THERAPY (RET) PRINCIPLES

Taming your Stymie Beasts involves changing the way you think about yourself and your weight-control challenge. This type of thinking usually includes a very elaborate internal dialogue. The quotes provided for each of the seven Stymie Beasts clearly illustrates such thinking. Every one of those dialogues created barriers to the key goal for weight controllers—developing a Healthy Obsession (defined in my prior books as "a sustained preoccupation with the planning and execution of target behaviors to reach a healthy goal"). You will learn a great deal more about healthy obsessions in Chapter 4. You learned about the cognitive biases that helped created and sustain the Stymie Beasts. So now, let's focus on removing those beastly barriers (illustrated below) by using Rational Emotive Therapy to transform the cognitive barriers into more constructive self-talk.

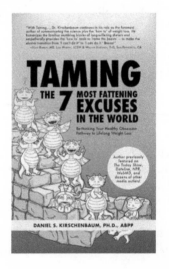

Certain types of irrational or problematic thoughts, like those in the Stymie Beasts' introductions, can easily prevent you from taking critical action steps. Let's consider Rational Emotive Therapy, or RET, now. RET is a very powerful way to help you shift your internal dialogues by modifying the way you think. More constructive actions can follow when you can tame the beasts in this way. You can even become undisturbable and extremely resilient in this way. Technically, "undisturbable" is not a word, but it's a great aspirational goal for those wanting to live a life with less distress. Developing the thinking skills that allow you to reach such lofty goals, however, takes some practice. This resembles most athletic challenges. If you can learn the way to think yourself to an undisturbable and resilient stance, then the payoff can take your weight-control game to a much higher level.

Shakespeare knew something about this:

> *"There's nothing either good or*
> *bad but thinking makes it so."*
> –William Shakespeare, *Hamlet*

INTRODUCTION TO **RET**

Psychologist Albert Ellis agreed with Shakespeare about this. Our thoughts powerfully influence our moods. In the 1950s, Dr. Ellis realized that the existing methods of helping people improve their moods, primarily psychoanalysis (a Freudian approach), did not work very well. He created a new approach based on analyzing the quality of thinking and how to change it. You will find using Ellis' Rational Emotive Therapy (RET) principles remarkably helpful. RET can help you change your biased thinking and, as a consequence, change your moods and actions and weight.

RET takes the position that the world and what we do in it/experience from it includes a series of positive, negative, and neutral events. Our thoughts interpret those events. Thoughts essentially create feelings, much more so than the actual events. If a weight controller saw the same number on a scale on Tuesday as Monday, then that weight controller might view that event as horrible and become very agitated (sad, frustrated). Another person in the exact same situation might consider that stability on the scale as a neutral or even positive event. The first weight controller expects weight losses perhaps every day. The second one knows that maintenance of weight beats gaining weight. Such feelings, in turn, can affect what we do (e.g., give up the weight control quest), which also can impact what we think (e.g., it's okay to quit trying). More generally, from an RET perspective, therefore, three response systems interact with each other constantly: thoughts, feelings, and behaviors.

STINKIN' THINKIN'

What kinds of thoughts make you sad or anxious? Think about the last time you felt either of those negative emotions. Can you trace backward from the emotions to the thoughts? Most people struggle to do that. Albert Ellis, Aaron Beck, and other theorists and researchers found that thoughts that decrease people's sense of hopefulness or control caused unhappy moods. They referred to such problematic thoughts as "irrational thoughts." Albert Ellis also called this "stinkin' thinkin'." Sometimes RET practitioners use the term "automatic thoughts" to describe this kind of stinkin' thinkin'. Take a look at the following examples and see if you can detect how and why thinking them could create problems:

- Everyone should love me.
- Every problem has an ideal solution.
- I have to be highly competent in everything I do.
- Other people should always treat me considerately and fairly.
- I must lose weight every week.
- If I don't lose weight every week, then I'm a failure—and I may as well give up.

- If I don't succeed every week, then my group leader and members will think I am worthless, a failure, and uncommitted; so, I may as well give up.
- If I don't eat the food my host offers me, she will hate me.
- I should not deprive my family of treats just because I am trying to lose weight.

What common elements did you observe in these irrational thoughts? Can you see the decreased sense of control some of them imply? For example, "I must lose weight ..." and "I have to be highly competent ..." demand a certain outcome with no wiggle room for alternatives. Some of these statements also engender hopelessness. The two statements that have "I may as well give up" at their conclusion certainly make that point clear.

The language within our thoughts provides cues that you can use to find your tendencies to think in problematic terms. Certain words tell the story. As I described it in my 2014 book on this subject, Table 3-1 summaries the types of extreme and absolute words that can help identify irrational or automatic problematic thoughts (APTs). Extreme words tend to exaggerate ideas and events, sometimes creating a sense of hopelessness. Absolute words, sometimes called "categorical imperatives," demand certain actions or outcomes. They tend to limit our sense of choice and control. Both hopelessness and feeling out of control can cause depressed or anxious feelings.

| EXTREME AND ABSOLUTE WORDS ||
Extreme Words	Absolute Words
All	Have to
Awful	Need
Essential	Must
Every	Ought
Horrible	Should
Terrible	
Totally	

TABLE 3-1

You can take several steps to examine the effects of these problematic thoughts in your life. First, try to go an entire day without using any of the absolute words listed in Table 3-1, both in what you say to others and also what you say to yourself. You will find it very challenging. Particularly try to avoid using the word "should" when talking to yourself or others. That's one of the most over-used and problematic words in the English language.

In order to give yourself a decent chance of succeeding at this challenge, it would help you to know the best alternatives to use. Try substituting an expression of preference or desire instead. For example, try to decide what you can say to modify the following statement to eliminate use of the word "should:" "Everyone should love me." Instead of "should," you can express a preference. For example, "I'd prefer it if everyone loved me, but I know that's impossible." Or, "I like it when people seem to like me, but I know that's not going to happen with everyone."

SEAT: Situation, Emotion, Automatic Problematic Thoughts, and Turn-Around Thoughts

Exercise 3-1 helps you track the use of these APTs and learn how to turn them around with alternative thoughts (TATs—Turn-Around Thoughts). Any time you experience a negative emotion for the next week, try entering it into this exercise and re-working your reaction to the situation that caused the APT. If you do this for several weeks, then you will take a huge step toward become more undisturbable. For additional examples, see the reprinted list of APTs below and the turn-around thoughts following each of them in italics. Then, try doing Exercise 3-1 over the course of the next week or weeks to practice these skills.

- Everyone should love me. *I'd like it if everyone loved me, but I know that's impossible. Some people just don't get along and that's okay.*
- Every problem has an ideal solution. *Problems, by definition, are challenges without immediately obvious or ideal solutions. Problems often have best solutions, but rarely do they have ideal solutions. For example, my car is getting older and starting to cost more and more money to keep running. I could get another car, but that's a huge expense. Or, I could keep sinking money into it and hope it keeps going for a while longer. Neither solution is ideal; both involve risks. If money was very tight, then keeping the car longer might make more sense; perhaps I'll make a decision after getting a mechanic I trust to give me his best guess as to the car's longevity.*
- I have to be highly competent in everything I do. *I'd like to be competent in everything, but that's unlikely. It also depends on my standards for competence. Is bowling 150 competent or does it take 200 consistently to reach that standard? It's*

just fine if I'm competent at the things that matter most to me and merely okay at others.

- Other people should always treat me considerately and fairly. *I'd like that to happen, but people vary tremendously in the way they treat each other. People also vary in the way they are likely to treat me based on how they feel on a particular day, their level of stress, and other factors.*

- I must lose weight every week. *As a weight controller, I'd like that. It's just unrealistic. So many factors determine the number on the scale. The scale is an imperfect measure of effort. I can control the effort I put into my program and my consistency in key areas, at least to some extent. It's harder to control a number on a scale.*

- If I don't lose weight every week, then I'm a failure—and I may as well give up. *I could use a much better standard to determine my success/failure than weight loss every week. For example, I can evaluate my consistency of self-monitoring and reaching my step goals. The process matters too, not just the numbers on the scale.*

- If I don't succeed every week, then my group leader and members will think I am worthless, a failure, and uncommitted; so, I may as well give up. *My group leaders and members are there to support me, not to reject me for being imperfect. They're not going to view me as worthless because I struggle at this difficult task. That would be both mean and unreasonable.*

- If I don't eat the food my host offers me, she will hate me. *Hosts don't care that much about what everyone eats. If someone were to hate me because of what I ate or didn't eat, then I wouldn't want her for a friend anyway.*

- I should not deprive my family of treats just because I am trying to lose weight. *My family wants to support me. The approach in this book allows for plenty of treats, just ones that are very low in fat and on the program. They'll learn to feel satisfied with those treats, and their health will improve because of this.*

SITUATION-EMOTION-AUTOMATIC PROBLEMATIC THOUGHTS—TURN-AROUND THOUGHTS (SEAT):

Changing Your Thinking to Improve Your Moods

Instructions: Use this form to track your negative emotions, identify the Automatic Problematic Thoughts (APTs) associated with them, and then use Turn-Around Thoughts (TATs) to decrease the negativity of those emotions. To do this:

1. Identify and then rate the EMOTION (E from the SEAT acronym). Use the following Subjective Unit of Discomfort Scale (SUDS) to do the rating: 0 = perfectly calm and happy to 100 = miserable beyond description, worst feeling possible.
2. Describe the SITUATION (S from SEAT).
3. Identify APTs (A from SEAT).
4. Write out TATs by re-writing the APTs in a more adaptive form (T from SEAT).

See the two examples in italics below the form and then complete the form with your own entries for this week.

SEAT WORKSHEET: SITUATION, EMOTION, APTs, TATs			
SITUATION: Day, Time, Happenings	**EMOTION, SUDS Rating**	**APTs: Automatic Problematic Thoughts**	**TATS: Turn Around Thoughts**

TABLE 3-1

SEAT Example			
SITUATION:	**Emotion & SUDS**	**Automatic Problematic Thoughts (APTs)**	**Turn Around Thoughts (TATs)**
Monday 9 a.m., got on my scale	Frustrated, 35	I **should** have lost weight this week.	I really wanted to lose weight and would have preferred losing weight this week. The scale is an imperfect measure. I know I worked at this because I self-monitored well and met my step goals.
Thursday 7 p.m., Friend's house for dinner	Annoyed/ Angry, 40	I **hate** when my friends offer me high-fat foods. It's a **horrible** bind that they put me in when they do that.	I'd rather my friends understood my weight control program better than they do; but this isn't a hateful act on their part. The bind I'm in is challenging, not horrible.

Using TUS and RET to Tame the Beasts

Let's revisit all seven of the Stymie Beasts and try to use both TUS and RET to thoroughly re-work the dialogue that emerged from them, all based on cognitive biases.

CAN'T

"I CAN'T LOSE WEIGHT. I'VE TRIED EVERYTHING; I'M JUST TIRED OF THE ROLLER COASTER—LOSE WEIGHT, FEEL GREAT GAIN IT ALL BACK, AND THEN SOME, AND FEEL LIKE CRAP. ALSO, I GAINED A LOT OF THIS WEIGHT BECAUSE OF A MEDICATION THAT I REALLY NEEDED, AND STILL NEED. LET'S FACE IT, I'VE TRIED EVERY DIET AND PROGRAM; NOTHING WORKS FOR ME. I'M DONE."

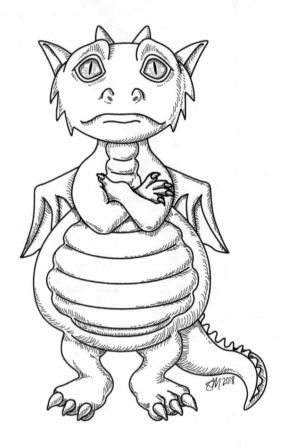

- "**I can't lose weight.**" The word "can't" itself suggests an absolute fact. It's not one of the absolute words listed in Table 3-2, in part because under some conditions it's a logical and accurate statement. For example, it's accurate to say:
  - I can't outrun the fastest person on the planet right now.
  - I can't rebuild my car's engine in the next ten minutes.
  - I can't fly.

These accurate statements stand in stark contrast to an overweight person claiming essentially that he or she cannot possibly lose weight. What if that person went to a prison that starved the prisoners? What if some benefactor agreed to pay that person $1,000,000 to lose ten pounds in the next month? How about this as a TAT: "I don't want to work at losing weight right now." That TAT allows for the possibility of finding a new approach and taking another shot at this healthy quest.

- "**I've tried everything ... I've tried every diet and exercise program.**" Which words make these statements fit the definition of APTs? "Everything" and "every" clearly exaggerate reality in extreme ways. Hundreds of diets and a host of programs exist. For example, in this book, we will discuss the concept of healthy obsession and the use of three primary dietary principles in the *Very Low Fat (VLF) Healthy Obsession Pathway (HOP)* (Chapters 4-8). Has the Can't Beast really tried this approach? What about a professionally conducted Cognitive Behavior Therapy (CBT) program, one you will read more about in subsequent chapters and the approach most recommended by expert groups? These latter points come from TUS perspective. The questions they raise include:

– How does what I have tried compare to what science tells us produces the best results?
– Can I get more effective help than the help/ approaches I have used before?

What's a good TAT to tame these exaggerated APTs? How about: "I have found it frustrating to try so many diets and programs and yet still have a weight problem. I know others exist and I could find some potentially better approaches if I were willing to work toward change."

• **"Nothing works for me."** "Nothing" makes it to the hit list as another APT. Clearly that's an exaggeration. How about this as a TAT: "Just because I haven't succeeded so far doesn't mean nothing can help me lose weight." Another TAT: "Nothing has worked for me yet. I have not as yet found something that works for me, but I'm sure it exists, and I can find it. If I look hard enough, then I will find a solution."

SUMMARY

CAN'T BEAST	
APTs: Automatic Problematic Thoughts	**TATS: Turn Around Thoughts**
I can't lose weight.	I don't <u>want</u> to work at losing weight right now.
I've tried everything.	I have found it frustrating to try <u>several diets and programs</u> and yet still have a weight problem. I know others exist and I could find some potentially better approaches if I were willing to work toward change.
Nothing works for me.	Just because <u>I have not succeeded so far,</u> that does not mean nothing can help me lose weight.

ADDICT

*"I HAVE TO HAVE MY CHOCOLATE FIX EVERY DAY, I JUST HAVE TO.
PEANUT BUTTER ALSO CALLS OUT TO ME EVERY DAY. I'VE TRIED
LOSING WEIGHT AND KNOW THAT WOULD BE A GOOD THING. I
JUST CAN'T GET PAST MY ADDICTION TO THESE CERTAIN FOODS. I'VE
COME TO JUST ACCEPT THAT AS PART OF MY REALITY."*

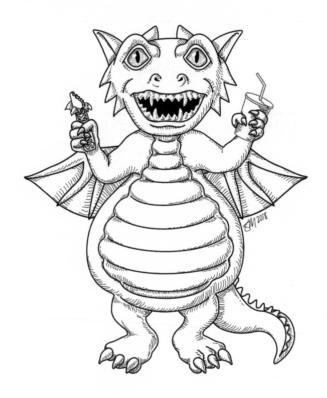

<u>COGNITIVE BIASES:</u> Affect, Confirmation, Outcome

- "I have to have my chocolate fix every day, I just have to." "Have to," repeated twice in this statement, appears prominently on the RET list of absolute words. It's a classic APT. How about this as a TAT: "Our hunter-gatherer ancestors no doubt survived for many centuries without a hint of chocolate. How could such a substance become a necessity when our ancestors did without it, as do many adults living today?" Another TAT: "Chocolate comes in very low fat and even lower calorie versions, like in yogurts and frozen yogurt and cocoa. I can find a way around this desired taste that doesn't hurt my efforts to lose weight."
- "I just can't get past my addiction to certain foods." "Can't" sits very close to "have to" among the list of RET absolutes. TAT for this one: "I'm struggling to get past my addiction to certain foods."
- "... addiction to certain foods." This one calls out, once again, for some TUS perspective: Does food addiction really exist or is it just another myth related to weight control? In my previous book, *Athlete, Not Food Addict*, I made a strong case, based on scientific evidence, that true food addictions happen to very few people. For example, look at the chart below that contrasts a respected definition of drug addiction (from the Diagnostic and Statistical Manual IV R– American Psychiatric Association) with supposed food addiction. Note the dramatic differences that testify to the myth of food addiction.

DRUG ADDICTS VS. OBESE PEOPLE		
	Drug Addicts	**Food Addicts???** **(Obese People)**
Distressed	Very frequently	Sometimes
Tolerance	Yes, most cases	No
Withdrawal	Yes, most cases	No
Loss of Control	Yes	Infrequently
Repeated Failures to Change	Yes	Yes, but isn't persistence at difficult tasks good?
Substantial Time to Obtain	Usually	No
Giving up Activities	Yes, frequently	Rarely
Sustained Use Despite Problems	Yes	Yes, but necessary for survival

For example, when people eat problematic food, they don't develop a tolerance for that food. One pint of high-fat Haggen-Das ice cream gobbled down today does not lead to longing for one and a half pints tomorrow. In the programs that I designed, Wellspring camps and boarding schools, about 10,000 participants switched in one day from their usual way of eating to eating very little fat and many fewer calories when they began their journeys in Wellspring. Not once did we send a teenager to the hospital for withdrawal symptoms. Such withdrawal quite simply never happened: Zero incidences out of 10,000 young people who attended Wellspring's programs (2004-2014).

Here's another important set of findings that dispute the usefulness of the food addiction notion. Clinicians and scientists who believe in food addiction believe that many or perhaps most overweight people who show clear signs of food addiction would really struggle to lose weight, much more than their non-addicted peers. After all, such food addicts would have strong cravings, uncontrollable binge eating, and other behaviors that would cause and maintain excess weight.

Two different groups of researchers tested this hypothesis in recent studies. In one case, overweight participants in weight loss programs who scored high on the Yale Food Addiction Scale did not predict outcomes better than a simple measure of binge eating. In a second and much larger study, world renowned weight management expert, University of Pennsylvania's Dr. Tom Wadden (a psychologist), and colleagues found that fifteen percent of their overweight adults scored high on that Yale Food Addiction Scale. These supposed food addicts, however, did just as well in a cognitive behavior therapy weight management program as their peers. The ostensibly addicted participants attended just as many sessions and lost just as much weight as their non-addicted peers over the entire six months of the study.

From a representative (TUS determined base rate) perspective, maybe one to three percent of people really suffer from food addiction to a significant degree. The Addict Beast exaggerates its desire to eat certain foods more than anything else, but is very unlikely to genuinely suffer from a food addiction. This desire to "have to" eat those high-fat foods exaggerates the reality of the situation. It's not like we have to eat chocolate to survive. If our hunter-gatherer ancestors could flourish without any chocolate, we can find a way to do so as well. Therefore, consider this:

TAT: "Food addiction is more myth than reality for almost everyone. I'm just finding it challenging to avoid eating some problematic foods."

SUMMARY:

ADDICT BEAST **SEAT** WORKSHEET: APTs, TATs	
APTs: Automatic Problematic Thoughts	**ATS: Turn Around Thoughts**
I have to have my chocolate fix every day, just have to	Our hunter-gatherer ancestors no doubt survived for many centuries without a hint of chocolate. How could such a substace become a necessity when our ancestors did without it, as do many adults living today?
I just can't get past my addiction to certain foods.	I'm struggling to get past my addiction to certain foods.
… food addict	Food addiction is more myth than reality for almost everyone. I'm just finding it challenging to avoid eating some problematic foods.

HATE

"There's nothing I hate more than exercising; well, maybe dieting. I just hate that feeling of pushing myself to move, sweating, getting tired, and wanting relief from all of that. I'm sort of amazed that anyone seems to like it. Maybe they're just masochists? Same thing with depriving myself of foods that I love. Where's the joy of living when you can't have beautiful tasty foods every day? It's just not for me. I agree with Mark Twain (echoed by Winston Churchill many years later), 'Whenever I get the urge to exercise, I lie down until the feeling passes away'."

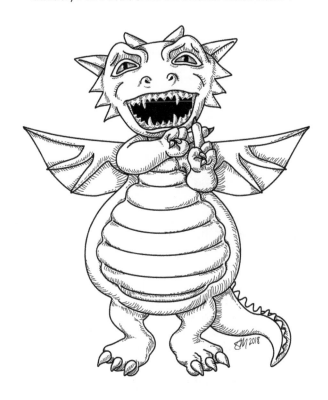

COGNITIVE BIASES: Affect, Recency

The Hate Beast's strong emotional reaction does not jive with the reality of the sort of movement required to lose weight or the possibilities for eating to lose weight. Invoking TUS here: Dozens of studies document the emotional benefits of movement. For example, see this figure below:

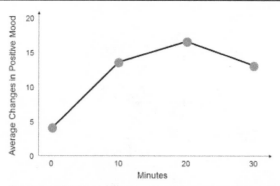

Hansen et al.(2001). Exercise duration and mood: How much does it take to feel better? Health Psychology, 20, 267-275.

This figure shows the results of a study published in a highly regarded peer-reviewed journal *(Health Psychology)* that found substantial emotional benefits from just ten minutes of walking. Movement generally improves moods and greatly improves overall health and well-being. That kind of movement can greatly improve weight management. Perhaps Hate Beast tried various strenuous exercise routines and found those too difficult. With some good research (TUS), it becomes apparent that any form of movement done consistently can aid weight control.

Training for marathons and lifting massive amounts of weight can be bypassed in favor of strolls in the park.

Similarly, one of the key eating principles I have espoused for many years (and echoed again later in this book in Chapter 6) encourages eating for pleasure, as well as successful weight control: Eat Likeable Foods That Like You Too. Can anyone who likes ice cream really "hate" frozen yogurt? Probably not. Can anyone who loves hot dogs really hate Hebrew National 97% Fat-Free Hot Dogs? Definitely not. Recipes abound on the internet for very low-fat versions of almost every food people really like, from chili to pizza to brownies. How does Hate Beast justify such distaste for such tasty foods? Perhaps a history of following unpleasant diets created a false impression of how to eat to maximize sustained success.

Some TATs that fit with this type of reasoning include:

- I can find plenty of likeable foods that like me too. I can just explore the possibilities and find them.
- Movement does not require intense, unpleasant work-outs. I can move to lose in ways that will make me healthier and happier.
- True—weight management requires discipline. A simple cost/benefit analysis shows that I can give it a good try using scientifically based approaches and may well benefit from that effort. I might even enjoy the process.

SUMMARY:

HATE BEAST SEAT WORKSHEET: APTs, TATs	
APTs: Automatic Problematic Thoughts	**TATS: Turn Around Thoughts**
I hate diet foods.	I can find plenty of likeable foods that like me too, like frozen yogurt instead of high fat ice cream.
I can't stand all of that exercising you have to do to lose weight.	Movement does not require incredibly intense workouts. I can move to lose in ways that will make me healthier and happier, like walking and listening to my favorite tunes along the way.
I hate all of that obsessively rigid discipline—makes me feel like I have no choices left in my life.	Weight control does require discipline, but I can learn to forgive myself for minor lapses and even enjoy the process. I can applaud good efforts and find plenty of choices in how I do it. Only I can make me feel trapped, not the process of losing weight.

LAZY

"I KNOW IT WOULD BE REALLY GOOD FOR ME TO LOSE THIS WEIGHT, BUT I'M JUST LAZY. I JUST DON'T LIKE PUSHING MYSELF TOO HARD AND I LOVE TO SLEEP, REST, AND JUST TAKE IT EASY. I WORKED HARD IN MY LIFE AND NOW I'M JUST TIRED OF THAT. I CAN'T SEEM TO GET TOO INTERESTED IN DOING WHAT IT WOULD TAKE TO LOSE WEIGHT."

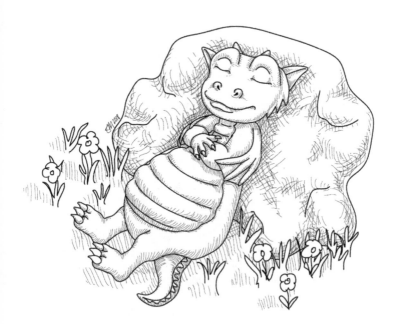

COGNITIVE BIASES: Affect, Recency

Invoking laziness actually means using a classic explanatory fiction. This Lazy Beast believes that laziness somehow explains an unwillingness to work toward change. How do you know if you're lazy? Many factors can impact the pursuit of change that have nothing to do with one's personality tendencies (i.e., laziness). Weight control does create inevitable frustrations, for example. Experience with such challenges can invoke the affect bias: making decisions based on feelings, not on TUS or logic. Also, the recency bias comes into play if recent efforts toward losing weight failed miserably. Failing recently can lead to believing success cannot happen, if that bias becomes activated.

Some examples of APTs associated with this Lazy Beast include:

- **I should not have to work hard at anything. That's just not fair anymore, after all I've been through in my life.** Notice the "should" statement leading off these two APTs. Also, the exaggeration word in that sentence: "anything." What about the concept of fairness invoked in the second sentence? Essentially: if you have worked hard in your life, then fairness dictates that you should not have to do that anymore?

  How about these TATs: It's understandable to prefer achieving progress without extremely hard work. Rather than say, "I should not have to work hard …", how about: "I'd prefer to find an easier, more comfortable way to lose weight than the methods I've tried in the past." Perhaps you, Lazy Beast excuse, did not find the most effective and efficient approach in the past. Science provides such an approach in VLF HOP that you will read about soon. How about giving that a shot this time around? After all, failure to pursue weight control creates lots of hard work too, including frequent doctor visits, relying on medications that have side effects, failing to live a long happy life, and other major costs for not pursuing this important goal.

Who determines what's fair in life? Is your body's resistance to weight loss inherently unfair? That's a bit like arguing that our body's relative slowness compared to most animals just is not fair. Our bodies evolved in a way that helps us have far more brain power than any other species. Is that unfair to dogs and cats? Biology just follows its own course, but we can use our big brains to manage it effectively, just as every athlete learns to do. So, the TAT here goes something like: "Life just is not fair. I will not allow a concept like absolute fairness in all things determine my life. I can work toward improving my life and I'm fortunate to have that chance."

- **"I love to sleep and rest and should be able to do as much of that as I like."** That "should" statement, if followed, would make just about everyone with a job late for work, taking naps whenever the tiredness felt noticeable, and resist working hard versus resting.
  It's great to love sleeping and rest. How does weight control prevent enjoyment of sleep and rest? It really doesn't do that, but it does demand effort.

So, the TATs here: "Achievement often requires effort, beyond just resting. Very few, if any, people get paid to rest as much as they might like. Work means going beyond the feeling of tiredness to reap such benefits as getting paid for your time and achieving success. Almost no one who succeeds in life expects to rest as much as they might like. They certainly don't follow some unwritten rule that promotes as much rest as possible or desired. Working for something

important, like health and well-being, provides many
important pay-offs—well worth the effort."

- **"I can't get interested in losing weight."** "Can't" …
or "won't"? "Can't"—an exaggerated word—suggests
that it's impossible to find a way to take the steps
necessary to lose weight. What if a benefactor offered a
million dollars to help those Lazy Beasts start counting
fat grams, steps, and working at losing weight? So,
consider these TATS: "I just have not as yet found a
way to make losing weight appealing. It's not that I
can't become motivated again; I just haven't found that
yellow brick road to make the path toward success
appealing again. I can get interested in weight loss, just
don't know how to spark that interest at the moment."

SUMMARY:

LAZY BEAST **SEAT** WORKSHEET: **APT**s, **TAT**s	
APTs: Automatic Problematic Thoughts	**TATS: Turn Around Thoughts**
I should not have to work hard at anything. That's just not fair.	I'd prefer to find an easier way to lose weight than the methods I've tried before. Life just isn't fair—and that's OK.
I should be able to sleep and rest as much as I like.	Achievement usually requires effort. People do not get paid to rest. Work means going beyond rest to get benefits—like payment and success.
I can't get interested in losing weight.	I just have not, as yet, found a way to make losing weight appealling again.

WON'T

"Losing weight just is not me. I can live a great life being big—and I'll stay healthy too. Several people in my family lived to be very old despite big waistlines. Some famous people did that too, like Alfred Hitchcock, 80; Aretha Franklin, 76; and Henry Kissinger, who is still writing political books at 93. Besides, I have a right to be big. In fact, I'm an advocate for the civil rights of fat people, just like my fellow members of the National Association to Advance Fat Acceptance (NAAFA)."

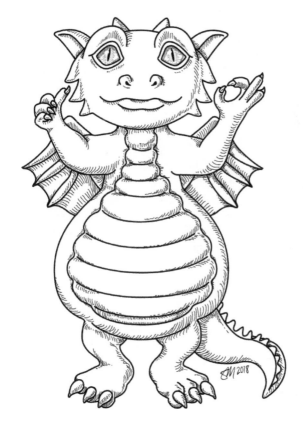

COGNITIVE BIASES: Representative, Confirmation, Overconfidence

"NAAFA is a non-profit, all volunteer, civil rights organization founded in 1969. NAAFA is dedicated to protecting the rights and improving the quality of life for fat people. NAAFA works to eliminate discrimination based on body size and provide fat people with the tools for self-empowerment through advocacy, education, and support. [Our vision is that we want] a society in which people of every size are accepted with dignity and equality in all aspects of life." https://www.naafaonline.com/dev2/about/

Cognitive biases play an especially major role for the Won't Beast. Most people, especially well-educated people, truly do use TUS to know the dangers of excess weight. Think about this: How many people do you know who would rely on representative bias to focus on Alfred Hitchcock as an example of the minimal impact of obesity? In other words, Hitchcock's relatively long life certainly doesn't accurately represent the evidence about the negative impact of excess weight. He was the rare exception, not the rule, based on TUS.

Confirmation bias in this case means that those with active Won't Beasts will look for evidence that supports this unusual stance. They will point out to friends and family that slim people sometimes die from heart attacks or cancer or other diseases, too. They will notice those overweight people around them who seem quite healthy. Conversely, when the obese star of the incredibly successful TV show *The Supranos,* James Gandolfini, died recently of a massive heart attack at 51, those who live with Won'ts will find another way of thinking about the cause of his premature death. They may think he just had a bad heart, not connecting that bad heart to his excess weight and lack of fitness.

Overconfidence bias also applies in this case, for many people. Believing in something so far removed from the scientific evidence requires a strong belief in distorted information—like the notion that they are likely to remain perfectly healthy despite their excess weight. Many arguments are lost on such people because they view their beliefs as unassailable truths. That overconfidence essentially builds a powerful wall that resists attacks from opposing forces using reason and TUS.

Consider these APTs often used by those plagued by Won't Beasts:

- **I'm perfectly healthy even though I'm obese, according to my doctor and the definition used by most people.** RET argues that extreme language creates emotional distress—such as the use of words like awful, horrible, and terrible. In this case, the extreme language of "perfectly healthy" creates a distortion of reality. TUS reasoning argues in favor of looking at science objectively. Widely available objective summaries of that science appear regularly in the newsletter from the Center for Science in the Public Interest, *Nutrition HealthLetter,* and from *Consumer Reports.*

  Obesity is objectively and most commonly defined by the Body Mass Index: Weight (kg)/Height $(m)^2$. Studies consistently show that BMI does correlate quite well with more direct measures of the amount of fat in the body. Those measures include underwater weighing (hydro-densitometry), Magnetic Resonance Imaging (MRI), and Computerized Tomography.

  If you want to check your current BMI, this website can help: https://www.cdc.gov/healthyweight/ assessing/bmi/adult_bmi/english_bmi_calculator/bmi_ calculator.html.

As indicated in Table 3-2, TUS shows that obesity, BMI above thirty for example, can contribute to more than a hundred different illnesses, many of which can become life-threatening. Tremendous increases in cost for individuals and societies have been documented as due directly to the worldwide obesity epidemic, as well. Some estimates show an increase in health care cost per obese person at about $10,000 per year. So, referring to oneself as "perfectly healthy" when excess weight makes that essentially impossible shows a willingness to ignore scientific reality.

DISEASES ASSOCIATED WITH OBESITY

High Blood Pressure   Cataracts

Heart Disease   Strokes

Lung Disease, especially Obstructive Sleep Apnea

Insomnia   Diabetes   High Cholesterol

Cancer (e.g., breast, colon, esophasgus, prostate

Gall Bladder Disease   Arthritis

Gynecologic abnormalities including intertility and Polysystic Ovarian Syndrome

Muscular skeletal disorders, including: Knees, hips, back and feet

Here's a TAT that could be useful in this regard:

"I wish my health was not affected by my excess weight. However, the scientific evidence indicates that even if I feel okay now, that won't sustain me in the long run. Life is a precious thing and I'm going to refocus on that."

- I hate the way people can be so mean to those
of us who are overweight. It's certainly true that
many negative stares and comments are made
every day about excess weight. Many hurtful
nicknames exist to describe overweight people: fat,
fatso, fatty, chubby, chunky, bulbous, porker, pig,
sow, whale, cow, blimp, and the list goes on. My
own nickname when I went to my first sleepaway
camp as an eight-year-old was "Chubsy." I really
hated that.
  But how does this negativity justify the Won't
approach to weight? The word "hate" provides a
strong clue regarding the irrationality of this stance.

  Here's a TAT that could help:
  "I dislike the negativity so many people express about
excess weight. I wish others could find a way to accept our
differences in size and just support efforts to get healthier.
That wish can happen with those close to me. I can use the
negativity as motivation to change, rather than just stew on it
and get entrenched in staying unhealthy (and overweight)."

- Being overweight has absolutely no effect on the
quality of my life, maybe with the exception of some
increased health risks in the long run. You can still
live a great life even with excess weight. That's true.
But effects of the excess weight, without a doubt,
include limiting options in many areas of life if you
use TUS to investigate it. Overweight (particularly
very overweight/obese) people are discriminated
against in seeking jobs and certainly get rejected
socially in most cultures. Employers, especially the
growing number of self-insured employers, don't
want the additional costs associated with excess
weight. As noted previously, some studies show
such costs can amount to an extra $10,000 per
year, as well as greater numbers of missed work

days due to illnesses. At least in most communities/
cultures, overweight people also get rejected more
so than normal weight folks as potential dates and
life partners.

Here's a TAT based on this analysis:

"Quality of life decreases when you get rejected at
higher rates due to excess weight from jobs and by
potential friends and lovers."

SUMMARY:

WON'T BEAST SEAT WORKSHEET: APTs, TATs	
APTs: Automatic Problematic Thoughts	**TATS: Turn Around Thoughts**
I'm perfectly healthy.	Perfect health rarely happens for overweight people. Healthy now does not translate to health as I get older.
I hate the way people get so mean to those of us with excess weight.	Hate can keep me from taking action to change, although disliking such negativity seems reasonable. It's tougher to change the culture than change myself.
Being overweight has absolutely no effect on the quality of my life, aside from some increased risk of illness.	Being overweight may not effect me much now, but it certainly can make finding the best job or best lover more difficult.

WAITING

"I KNOW MY MOTIVATION WILL KICK IN AGAIN. I CAN FEEL IT. I LOST 75 POUNDS JUST THREE YEARS AGO. I WAS SO GUNG HO— NOTHING COULD GET IN MY WAY THEN. SOMETHING JUST GRABBED ME AND MOTIVATED ME FOR MONTHS AND MONTHS. I'M JUST WAITING FOR IT TO COME BACK AGAIN—AND I KNOW IT WILL."

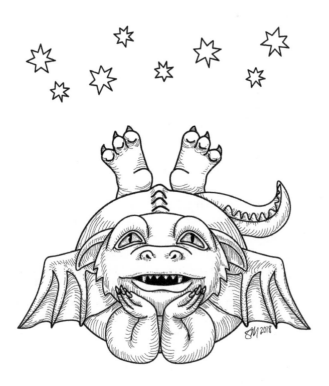

COGNITIVE BIAS: Representative, Outcome, Availability, Conservatism, Overconfidence

- **I know for sure my motivation will just kick in again if I wait long enough.** Many factors combine to motivate change, some of which are quite particular to certain moments in time/place. For example, weight controllers report gearing up for this effort due to medical crises, difficulty wearing a particular pair of pants, successful weight loss by a friend, suddenly having the time to focus on exercise, and many other factors. Note that none of these motivators resembles some special internal state that just shows up to get people to spring into action. One thing the extensive research on cognitive biases makes super clear (a TUS conclusion): we cannot trust our usual thought processes when trying to understand how we think. We're subject to a host of cognitive biases in the way we think.

    TAT: "Our internal motivational state can change at any time due to a host of external influences. Therefore, knowing 'for sure' that your motivation will kick in is delusional; it may never happen."

- **I won't be able to change unless I'm really motivated to change.** What if someone offered you $1,000,000 right now to self-monitor everything you eat, eat no more than ten fat grams per day, and walk 20,000 steps per day—and to do this every single day for a hundred days? Would you do it? Motivation comes from many sources. Building momentum toward an important goal can completely alter your perspective, regardless of how you got there. Sometimes just following a good scientifically based approach can lead to changes in behavior and outcomes, even without any detectable change in the inner drive or dialogue.

TAT: "Change can occur through a great many avenues, which in turn can lead to positive outcomes, even without a major alteration in internal states. Motivation is dynamic—impacted by what we do sometimes more than how we think about things."

- **In these modern times, we all seem to rush into everything, usually getting nothing in return.** Certainly, rushing into making key decisions can lead to troubling impulsive outcomes—like buying the wrong car or taking the wrong job. However, very few of us rush into everything. Also, sometimes just doing something that seems appealing leads to excellent outcomes—networking, finding out interesting things, and just having fun.

TAT: "Making quick choices can sometimes produce great outcomes, especially if such choices come from studying reliable sources of information (like TUS-driven reviews of Consumer Reports). Those outcomes far exceed 'nothing.' Speed of decision making does not necessarily reflect or cause poor decision making." Certainly not all of us rush decision making; maybe some of us do so some of the time.

SUMMARY:

WAITING BEAST SEAT WORKSHEET: APTs, TATs	
APTs: Automatic Problematic Thoughts	**TATS: Turn Around Thoughts**
I know my motivation will kick in again if I wait long enough.	Internal motivation states can change due to lots of external factors. You cannot know for sure that it will ever happen just by waiting.
I won't change unless I'm really motivated.	Change can occur through many means, not just via internal changes first. Motivation is dynamic, affected more by what we do than what we think.
We seem to rush into everything and often get nothing in return.	Very few of us rush into "everything." And, quick well-informed decisions can lead to great outcomes—far from "nothing."

HOW?

"I really want to succeed, but I just don't know how to do it. I've tried lots of things and I still believe something out there will work for me. I keep trying the latest and what seems like the best ideas, but no luck yet. I'm just searching for that and I refuse to give up. I know people have succeeded in losing weight and keeping it off. Why not me, too?"

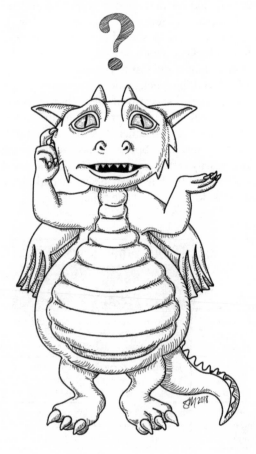

Innovation, Anchoring, Availability

- **I keep trying the latest and greatest diets, but not succeeding with them.** This thinking reveals the incredible importance of TUS to taming the Stymie Beasts. Let's consider how science works. It provides clearly described, objective methodology to test solutions to well-defined problems. Those attempts then are published in peer-reviewed journals, if they succeeded to some reasonable degree.

  In contrast to scientifically derived solutions, the "latest and greatest" usually translates to approaches simply marketed as such. For example, a current trend that appears in many bestsellers advocates for eating only whole foods, no processed foods, and for fasting or nearly fasting a couple of days per week.

  Dr. Jennifer Poti and several of her colleagues from the University of North Carolina-Chapel Hill recently analyzed food purchases from more than 150,000 households from 2000-2012. They found that about seventy-seven percent of the foods we eat meet the usual definitions of moderately or highly processed foods. Where's the science that says eliminating seventy-seven percent of the foods we usually eat can really help us lose weight? This approach would eliminate eating such things as fat-free cheese, ninety-nine percent fat-free ground turkey, baked beans, frozen yogurt, and veggie burgers. Why in the world would eating such foods create problems for weight controllers?

  We used such foods every single day in Wellspring, producing some of the best results ever reported (in many peer-reviewed articles in scientific journals) for any weight loss program. The graph below helps make that point. Notice the dramatic weight losses for participants after camp and at follow-up, especially compared to where they likely would have been if they did not attend camp (i.e. trajectory of weight gain likely to affect them at the follow-up time period). Doesn't going from about seventy percent overweight before camp to about forty percent overweight a year later seem much better than going from seventy percent overweight to perhaps seventy-five percent overweight a year later?

WELLSPRING RESULTS: TWO YEARS OF FOLLOW-UPS

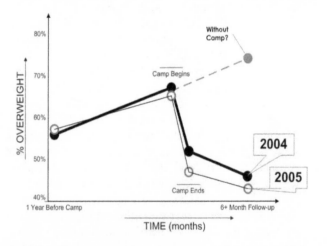

Reprinted, with permission from Mary Ann Liebert, Inc. Publishers: Kirschenbaum, D.S., Craig, R.D., Kelly, K.P., & Germann, J.N. (2007). Immersion programs for treating pediatric obesity: Follow-up evaluations of Wellspring Camps and Academy of the Sierras – A boarding school for overweight teenagers. Obesity Management, 3, 261-266.

Nothing that has appeared in peer-reviewed scientific journals supports using an approach like eliminating all processed foods, especially when compared to the Very Low-Fat Healthy Obsession Pathway presented later in this book. HOP, which is very similar to the approach Wellspring used from 2004-2014, yields very encouraging outcomes.

The same goes for fasting. That's another type of radical unscientifically based approach, very difficult to do, and generally produces excessive eating on subsequent days.

To accentuate this point about the serious misdirection provided by many new and popular approaches, let's consider ten recent bestsellers in the diet/weight loss category. I selected the following books by reviewing bestsellers in 2017 from the New York Times "Food and Diet" list and Amazon's "Diets and Weight Loss" bestsellers list:

- Davis, W. (2011). *Wheat Belly*. NY: Rodale.
- Dispirito, R. (2016). *The Negative Calorie Diet*. NY: Harper Collins.
- Fung, J. (2016). *The Obesity Code*. Vancouver, Canada: *Greystone*.
- Gundry, S.R. (2008). *Dr. Gundry's Diet Evolution*. NY: Harmony/Random House.
- Hartwig, D., & Hartwig, M. (2012). *It Starts with Food*. Las Vegas, NV: Victory Belt.
- Hartwig, M., & Hartwig, D. (2015). *The Whole 30*. NY: Houghton Mifflin Harcourt.
- Hyman, M. (2016). *Eat Fat, Get Thin*. NY: Little Brown.
- Pomroy, H. (2012). *The Fast Metabolism Diet*. NY: Harmony/Random House.
- Stork, T. (2016). *The Lose Your Belly Diet*. Los Angeles, CA: Ghost Mountain.
- Vogel, L. (2017). *The Keto Diet*. Las Vegas, NV: Victory Belt.

COMPARISONS OF THE PRESENT BOOK TO TEN BESTSELLERS ON SEVERAL KEY EMPHASES IN WEIGHT LOSS BOOKS

	Healthy Obsession	Healthy Obsession Defined	Maximize Movement-Track Steps	Self-Monitor	Self-Mon. Vital
Taming the 7 Most Fattening Excuses in the World	✔	✔	✔	✔	✔
Davis, *Wheat Belly*	X	X	X	X	X
DiSpirito, *Negative Calorie Diet*	X	X	X	X	X
Fung, *Obesity Code*	X	X	X	X	X
Gundry, *Diet Revolution*	X	X	X	X	X
D. Hartwig, *Starts With Food*	X	X	X	X	X
M. Hartwig, *Whole 30*	X	X	X	X	X
Hyman, *Eat Fat, Get Thin*	X	X	X	X	X
Pomroy, *Fast Metabolism*	X	X	X	X	X
Stork, *Belly Diet*	X	X	✔	X	X
Vogel, *Keto Diet*	X	X	X	X	X

TABLE 3-3

Table 3-3 summarizes some remarkable facts about the ten recent bestsellers. None of them even mentions the key phrases "healthy obsession" and "self-monitoring." Healthy obsession is a type of sustained focus on the key target behaviors necessary for success in weight management, as you will see in more detail in a subsequent chapter. I first coined that term in 1994, and since then, TUS tells us that quite a few studies have used that phrase when describing successful lifestyle changes in weight control.

Self-monitoring, the systematic observation and recording of target behaviors to reach a goal, has been described by Dr. Tom Wadden (one of the most widely acclaimed psychologists in the world specializing in weight management) as the "cornerstone" of cognitive-behavior therapy approaches to lose weight. Research on self-monitoring dates back to the early 1970s and has been included in numerous studies since then in top journals and books, easily meeting TUS criteria. In addition, every researcher and clinician who knows the science of weight loss stresses the importance of physical activity. Yet only one of the ten bestsellers even mentions maximizing movement by setting goals and self-monitoring steps (Stork, 2016).

Scientifically sound approaches to losing weight appear in professional journals and books written by scientists, but non-scientists struggle to find and understand such materials. Fortunately, as mentioned previously, at least two resources that don't accept commercial advertising summarize those important studies regularly:

- *Consumer Reports Magazine* (available digitally or in print); and, 2. Center for Science in the Public Interest's *Nutrition Action HealthLetter* (also available electronically or in print).

    TAT: "Latest" and "greatest" usually means the most well-advertised recent approaches. Those well-marketed approaches rarely translate into science. Instead, they just promote something that could make the originator money. Science provides the better alternatives, not advertised in a flashy widely available way, but still accessible to all who are willing to look carefully for it.

- **I have not been lucky in my efforts to lose weight.** Does luck sound like a scientifically based approach to you? Luck implies a good fortune determined by chance. TUS thinking tells us that science decreases solutions that solve problems based on chance by systematically testing hypotheses and developing empirically based models/theories.

  TAT: Science can work far better than luck. Remember Mark Twain's (echoed by baseball superstar Willie Mays) saying about luck: "The harder I work, the luckier I get." Systematic and scientifically based efforts generally produce far better outcomes than those based on chance (luck).

- **I keep looking for something new and exciting to motivate me.** Does newness yield the best outcomes? TUS shows that a very low-fat diet, lots of movement, and consistent self-monitoring works better than any new approach. Simply put, new doesn't mean better. Coca-Cola created a new type of Coke many years ago. They quickly had to re-issue "Coke Classic" because many Coke drinkers disliked the new version of Coke.

  In another TUS example, Consumer Reports recently (October 2017) recommended against buying newly revised models of pretty much every car. They argued that their data suggests that new often means worse in new cars. After a year or so, the problems in the revised version of a car generally get figured out and fixed, but it seems to take that year-plus to yield more reliable versions of most cars.

  Success breeds success—and motivation. TUS validated approaches breed such success.

TAT: New does not mean better; sometimes it means worse. Success breeds success—and that comes mostly from scientifically proven approaches.

SUMMARY:

How Beast SEAT Worksheet: APTs, TATs	
APTs: Automatic Problematic Thoughts	**TATS: Turn Around Thoughts**
I keep trying the latest and greatest diets, but failing with them all.	"Latest" and "greatest" usually means well-advertised fads, not scietifically validated methods. Science works better than fads.
I've been unlucky in my efforts to lose weight.	Science provides direction for efforts. Luck means leaving it up to chance. Remember, the harder you work (particularly following systematically tested and published pathways), the luckier you'll get.
I keep looking for something new and exciting to motivate me to change.	New does not guarantee better; sometimes it means worse. Success breeds success— and science breeds success.

SUMMARY AND CONCLUSION

Table 3-3 summarizes the nature of all seven Stymie Beasts, and the bottom line used to tame them. These Beasts develop over many years in most cases, and they defend their positions with considerable fortitude, despite their development from cognitively biased thinking. Once you identify the Beasts impacting you, you can start taming them and moving forward toward permanent success. TUS and RET approaches can break down the barriers that the Beasts create, unleashing great possibilities for positive change. Now, it's time to learn what really causes excess weight (HOP Step 1), and the four other simple but challenging HOP steps (2-5) you can take to move toward lifelong weight control.

SUMMARY OF STYMIE BEASTS AND KEY TAMING THOUGHTS

Stymie Beasts	Stymie Thoughts	Taming Thoughts
	CAN'T: I've tried every diet, and nothing works for me. I'm done!	Just because you haven't succeeded so far does not mean that you cannot find a new way to lose weight. You have not yet tried the type of cognitive behavior therapy approach (VLF HOP's five steps) featured in this book. You can do this, if you give science a real chance to help you.
	ADDICT: I just can't get past my addiction to food.	Food addiction is more myth than reality. You're just finding it tough to avoid certain problematic foods — and to succeed at the substantial challenge of weight control.
	HATE: There's nothing I hate more than exercising; well, maybe dieting.	You can find plenty of lovable foods that work well on this program. You can also learn to enjoy the many benefits of movement without forcing yourself to train for a marathon. Achieving some success will help quiet the hate.

	LAZY: I know it would be good to lose weight, but I'm just too lazy.	The CBT program in this book makes losing weight easier and more likely to happen. Success will energize you; you can use that energy to strive toward even more success.
	WON'T: Losing is just not me. I can live a great life being big.	TUS makes it clear that your "great life" will become much more painful, expensive, and shorter (i.e., not so great anymore) if you give up on losing weight—and stay overweight.
	WAITING: I know my motivation will kick in again. I'm just waiting for it to come back.	Motivation is dynamic, capable of changing more by what you do than what you think. You can start working toward change by following this program—starting right now.
	HOW? I really want to succeed, but I just don't know how. I keep searching for the "latest and greatest" approach.	Time to use TUS to see and believe in HOP's five steps in this book. Science works far better than fads. Success breeds success—and science breeds success.

TABLE 3-3

PART II

The VLF Healthy Obsession Pathway (HOP) in Five Steps

CHAPTER 4
Losing Weight Permanently

HOP Step 1: Understanding the Causes of Excess Weight

We will consider the primary causes of weight problems and then consider how best to fix them. You will benefit from knowledge of your challenges, similar to athletes who benefit from knowing the details of how to master their sports. The accomplished tennis player knows her equipment, from rackets to shoes to court surfaces. All elite athletes understand the requirements of their training regimens. Masterful weight controllers benefit by learning the causes of weight gain and the best approaches to lose weight.

Before focusing specifically on weight control, some discussion of psychology—the science of behavior— seems worthwhile, especially from a TUS perspective. Understanding psychological principles, or factors that predict and control behavior more generally, will help you create a foundation of knowledge to help frame the presentation about weight loss. Every sport has fundamentals. For example, a well-known instructor and late and great friend of mine, Dr. DeDe Owens, described the three fundamentals of the golf swing as grip, posture, and pivot (or how a golfer turns away from the ball to generate power). When golfers struggle with their swings, they go back to those three fundamentals to figure out the cause of the problem and the fix for it.

Psychology provides the fundamental knowledge required to understand how and why people gain and lose weight in much the same way.

PSYCHOLOGY: FACTORS THAT IMPACT BEHAVIOR, INCLUDING BEHAVIOR CHANGE

THREE RESPONSE SYSTEMS. Consider any complex behavior or emotion, like anxiety. What occurs to you when you think about the last time you felt anxious? Maybe you had to give a talk to colleagues. Maybe you had to make a five-foot putt to win a hole, or confront a boss or loved one about a problem. Try describing that anxiety. You could describe it in terms of behaviors, like saying "Uh" frequently or moving around in a jittery way. You could also describe the feeling itself. Anxiety feels unpleasant, queasy, or uneasy. You could also describe thoughts, like doubting yourself or worrying or expecting problems and more unpleasantness. Finally, anxiety often has a biological response or two like excess sweating, breathing rapidly, and elevated heart rate.

Psychologist Peter Lang did a series of landmark studies showing that the three response systems pictured in Figure 4-1 function in a related way during emotional reactions, but also quite independently at times. Someone giving a speech, for example, may look calm to the audience, but report afterwards tremendously unpleasant feelings and thoughts. The calm behavior in this case occurred independently from the thoughts and feelings. This applies directly to weight control. Some weight controllers may eat problematic foods, in quantities beyond their goals, and report feeling unconcerned about that deviation from the plan. Others react with tremendous negative emotion when drifting away from plans and goals. It helps to know that when thinking about approaches to losing weight, some or all three response systems can impact the outcome of the effort.

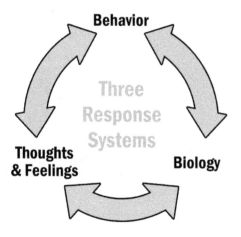

Reprinted, with permission, from May Ann Liebert, Inc., publisher: Kirschenbaum, D.S. (2010). Weight loss camps in the US and the Immersion-to-Lifestyle Change model. *Childhood Obesity*, 6, 318-323.

FIGURE 4-1. THREE RESPONSE SYSTEMS
FUNCTION SOMEWHAT INDEPENDENTLY.

BIOLOGICAL, SOCIAL-ENVIRONMENTAL, AND INTRA-PERSONAL DETERMINANTS OF BEHAVIOR. Figure 4-2 shows that these three factors influence our behaviors in powerful ways. Biology affects us every day. For example, our genetics impact our height, skin color, personality, and our tendency to gain weight easily. The culture in which we live affects us, too. As Americans, most of us have more than enough money and access to stores and restaurants that we can easily buy high quality, very low-fat foods, or also high-fat, problematic foods. Clearly family and friends impact us, too. If we have very active athletic families and friends, getting and staying active becomes a natural and ingrained part of our lifestyles. Sedentary friends and family can affect us in the opposite direction. Finally, we also have active inner (or intra-personal) lives.

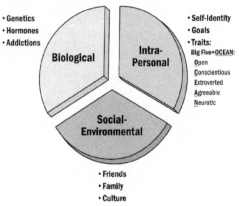

• Genetics
• Hormones
• Addictions

Biological

Intra-Personal

• Self-Identity
• Goals
• Traits:
Big Five=OCEAN:
Open
Conscientious
Extroverted
Agreeable
Neurotic

Social-Environmental

• Friends
• Family
• Culture

FIGURE 4-2. THREE MAJOR INFLUENCES ON BEHAVIOR:
BIOLOGICAL, SOCIAL-ENVIRONMENTAL AND INTRA-PERSONAL.

Those who favor a view of weight controllers as food addicts greatly over-emphasize our intra-personal lives. These food addict advocates essentially argue that emotional problems cause overweight people to binge eat to cope with the stresses of life. That ignores the biological realities of obesity such as genetic factors, and cultural influences such as the over-abundance of cheap heavily advertised high-fat foods on every street corner.

Our identities and goals also impact us. Think of the most athletic people you know. When such people describe themselves, they immediately start talking about their sports with big smiles on their faces. Weight controllers can either set goals to change, or not. For example, research shows that when people wear pedometers to measure their steps, those that also set goals (like 10,000 steps per day) record significantly more steps on average than those who do not set specific goals.

Personality traits are relatively enduring characteristics that affect our behaviors and attitudes in certain ways in many situations. Psychologists Paul Costa and Robert McCrae (at the National Institutes of Health) and Lewis Goldberg (at the University of Oregon) discovered that five broad dimensions of personality seem to work well to describe our general tendencies to behave in predictable ways. Called the Big Five, the researchers figured this out by asking thousands of people hundreds of questions, and then analyzing the data with a statistical procedure (factor analysis) that grouped the responses into their simplest form. The Big Five has become the most widely accepted model of personality by researchers.

The acronym OCEAN summarizes the names of the Big Five: Openness to Experiences, Conscientiousness, Extraversion, Agreeableness, and Neuroticism (emotional instability). Complete Exercise 4-1 to see the defining terms for each of the Big Five, and also to get an estimate of your Big Five tendencies. You can certainly score high on one or several of these traits.

EXERCISE 4-1: BIG FIVE PERSONALITY TEST

Based on a brief version of a questionnaire about the Big Five personality traits by Samuel Gosling and colleagues at the University of Texas, answer the ten questions below. Use the following seven-point rating scale to answer the questions:

1 = Disagree Strongly, 2 = Disagree, 3 = Disagree Somewhat, 4 = Neither Agree nor Disagree, 5 = Agree Somewhat, 6 = Agree, 7 = Agree Strongly

I see myself as:
1. Extraverted, socially dominant, full of enthusiasm.
2. NOT shy or reserved.
3. NOT overly critical and argumentative.
4. Sympathetic and warm.
5. Open to new experiences

6. Unconventional and creative
7. Well organized, careful, and responsible.
8. Dependable and self-disciplined.
9. Emotionally unstable
10. Easily upset, sometimes anxious or depressed.

High scores on the following items suggest tendencies toward the trait listed before them: Extraverted: 1 and 2; Agreeable: 3 and 4; Open: 5 and 6; Conscientious: 7 and 8; Neurotic: 9 and 10.

Several remarkable studies show that one of these traits in particular predicts weight status decades after people complete personality tests such as the brief one in Exercise 4-2. Which one do you think predicts relatively lower weights over time? If you guessed conscientiousness, then you got it right. Dr. Sarah Hamson and her colleagues reported a forty-year follow-up study conducted in Hawaii. Teachers assessed the Big Five traits of 753 ten-year-old children; then forty years later, health professionals measured a variety of things. Those people the teachers rated low in conscientiousness as ten-year-olds tended to have higher blood pressure, higher cholesterol, and higher Body Mass Indexes (a standard measure of weight divided by height). People who generally tend to persevere in the face of challenges, completing tasks in disciplined and well-organized ways, seem to manage their health better than people who score high on other traits.

CAUSES OF EXCESS WEIGHT

Understanding the three response systems (behavior, thoughts and feelings, biology) and the three primary influences on behavior (social-environmental, biological, and intra-personal) sets the stage for delving into the causes of excess weight gain. Let's consider the possible causes of weight problems from that perspective, including an analysis of the social-environmental factors and the other influences we just reviewed.

The "Obesogenic" Environment

About ten years ago, experts began referring to our culture as "obesogenic." This means that it has become the natural response to our social environment, and the culture of most developed countries, to gain excess amounts of weight over time. Our social environment essentially nurtures obesity, even encourages it. Let's review some highlights of this crazy culture:

- *Super-size me.* A traditional burger, fries, and Coke at McDonald's used to contain 627 calories and 19 grams of fat. Today, the standard combo (with a large order of fries, double cheeseburger, large drink) has 1,805 calories and 84 grams of fat— nearly triple the calories and more than quadruple the fat! A standard serving of Coca-Cola used to be 6.5 oz.—90 calories. Today, the standard serving is 20 oz. and packs 250 calories. There used to be only one size Snickers bar—1.1 oz., or 210 calories. Today, the Snickers "Big One"—3.7 oz.—more than doubles that with 500 calories.

Why have portions been super-sized? Like all companies, food and beverage companies—packaged goods and restaurants alike—aim to maximize their profits. And over the past generation, they realized that they can make more money through larger portions. If you're McDonald's and you charge $1.19 for small fries and $1.79 for large fries, which item will make you the most money? The large fries, versus the small, includes a slightly larger box and the additional potatoes and oil. Those elements probably cost McDonald's a penny or less per serving more than the small fries. Yet you charge the customer an extra sixty cents; that's almost pure profit. The overhead (the physical restaurant itself), the franchise fee, the labor, electricity—

all of these costs are the same regardless of whether the customer buys a small or a large. So, if you're McDonald's, your profit goes way up when you sell super-sized portions. Unfortunately, many people seem to value more food for their dollar, viewing it as a good deal. In fact, the company benefits from this good deal substantially. It's a bad deal for us.

- *Out to lunch.* With our fast-paced lifestyle, we're also eating more and more meals away from home, prepared by someone else. In 1975, Americans ate twenty-five percent of their meals outside of the home. Today, Americans probably eat out about fifty percent of the time. Restaurant meals account for about fifty cents out of every dollar Americans spend on food—almost half of which is spent at fast-food eateries.

Eating out is convenient. It's fun. But the tradeoff is control. By going out to eat, we're giving up control of ingredients, method of preparation, and portion size. As very few restaurants put your weight and health at the top of their agendas, you make compromises on each of these dimensions when you eat out. You wouldn't make those compromises if you ate at home and retained control.

- *Advertising.* Food and beverage companies try to generate good returns for their shareholders. It turns out a good way to do that has been to market large portions of high-fat, calorie-dense foods to us and to our children. Food and beverage marketers spend over fifteen billion dollars per year in the US and Canada, promoting their products just to children and teens. Most of these ads show junk food in colorful packaging that appeals quite a lot to children. And it works. Multiple studies have shown that children who are exposed to advertising ask their parents to buy high-fat, calorie-dense foods and sugary beverages. It's what kids want. It's what they pester you to buy. It's what they buy themselves. In their remarkable 2004 book Food Fight, Drs. Kelly Brownell and Katherine Horgen pointed out a basic inequity:

> "At its peak, the Five-A-Day fruit and vegetable program from the National Cancer Institute had $2 million for promotion. This is one-fifth the $10 million used annually to advertise Altoids mints."

It's simply not a level playing field.

Advertising for soft drinks in the US alone has increased much faster in recent years than other advertising, going from $541 million in 1995 to $800 million in 1999—an almost fifty percent increase in four years. In the past generation, the percentage of American children who drink soda increased from thirty-seven percent to over sixty percent, and average daily consumption among children who drink soda increased from 14 to 21 ounces. Researchers correlated amount of exposure to ads with a reduction in consumption of fruits and vegetables, presumably corresponding to an increase in the consumption of less nutritious foods. Every additional hour of television per day results in one less serving of fruits and vegetables every six days.

- *School Daze.* Another important factor is the near elimination of physical education in most school districts. Forced to focus on reading and math test scores by federal and state governments, but with no more time in the school day, and few more resources, school officials cut electives like art, music, and physical education. Today, only eight percent of American elementary schools, six percent of middle schools, and five percent of high schools provide daily physical education.
- *New World Living.* In the US and Canada, only ten percent of city travel occurs outside of cars, buses,

or trains. In relatively newer cities, like Los Angeles, Atlanta, and Dallas, where people rely on cars for almost everything, fewer than five percent of trips involve biking or walking. In contrast, people bike or walk at least forty percent in urban areas of Austria, Denmark, the Netherlands, and Sweden. People travel by bike or walk for at least thirty percent of their urban trips in France, Germany, and Switzerland.

Some of this change is due to where we're living. More Americans and Canadians now live in suburbs and so-called "exurbs" than ever before. Between 1970 and 2000, the percentage of Americans living in suburbs or exurbs grew from thirty-eight percent to fifty percent. In the past fifty years, suburbs accounted for ninety percent of the growth in US metropolitan areas. People drive far more in such areas, and builders now often avoid even laying down sidewalks in new developments.

Suburban and exurban living has its benefits, but physical activity isn't one of them. Suburban dwellers weigh on average six pounds more than those who live in cities. Researchers have also connected time spent driving with obesity—the odds of being obese increase six percent with each hour per day spent in the car.

- *Being Sane in Insane Places.* This phrase, captures the quest for healthy living in modern developed cultures. We get bombarded with ways of eating too much of the wrong kind of food and with appealing sedentary activities. Every new electronic gadget filled with apps enables us to do more by moving less. Every party and celebration includes so many caloric excesses that it becomes difficult to navigate life without developing excess weight. Our obesogenic culture wins far more than it loses these days.

Other Causal Elements: Biology, Psychology, Family, and Education

Let's start with this question: *What makes losing weight and keeping it off so difficult?*

Most people answer this question by invoking challenges like fast food, texting, super-sized portions, and busy lifestyles. Although these factors certainly contribute to the problem, what is the chief culprit? If you had to pick one primary factor that causes weight problems more than any other, what would you say? More specifically, try answering the second part of this question: *What makes losing weight and keeping it off so difficult? Is it biology or everything else?*

Biology in this case means genes (inherited tendencies), fat cells, hormones, enzymes, and metabolic rates (the amount of energy your body requires to simply stay alive at rest). "Everything else" refers to culture, family influences, habits, lifestyles, personality, and emotional functioning. Both biology and everything else clearly influence weight. But, if you had to pick one as your primary culprit, which one would you select? Does biology or does everything else have the most powerful impact on your weight?

If you answered like ninety-five percent of people to whom I've posed this question, you would say that both answers were correct, but that "everything else" clearly has the edge over "biology." This is the logical answer. After all, the environment, culture, and our habits and lifestyle seem to be responsible for weight gain. But that perfectly logical and reasonable answer isn't the best one.

It turns out it's biology that makes losing weight and keeping it off so difficult, even more than "everything else." Research by Canadian psychologist Claude Bouchard at Laval University helped make this point. Dr. Bouchard and his colleagues studied twelve sets of young male identical twins who lived in a controlled environment for a hundred days. After a baseline period of twelve days, the twins were given 1,000 calories above their usual levels of intake for the next eighty-four days. Some participants gained about nine pounds. but others gained almost thirty pounds—all under virtually identical conditions. The best predictor of how much weight any one boy gained was how much his twin gained. Some twins apparently had the biological tendency to gain weight easily, whereas others did not.

If you fully understand the power of biology as a cause of this problem, you will appreciate why becoming a successful weight controller demands considerable effort and support. Weight controllers have to learn what is and what isn't okay for them at home and when eating out. In sharp contrast, those who don't have this biological handicap don't ever have to think about it.

Developing an understanding of these biological challenges can help you start down the path of long-term weight control. This understanding begins by considering the biological demands faced by our collective ancestors.

Our Hunter-Gatherer Bodies

Let's take an imaginary trip back in time. Experts tell us that somewhere between 7,000 to 10,000 years ago, humans began farming, raising crops, and keeping animals. Try to imagine what life was like in the 200,000 to 300,000 years before that happened, when the first people who had bodies very much like ours were born.

- We would wake up in a different place every day because, without domestic animals or crops, we would have to search for food.
- We would be members of a tribe of ten to twenty people, each depending on each other for survival.
- You would pull out your smart phone made of stone and see only two words: *"Stay alive!"*
- You saw those the same words yesterday, the day before, and the year before. In fact, we would all be focused on four goals: find food, find shelter, raise our families, and most of all, stay alive.

- Look around at your fellow tribe members. Everyone would be muscular from years of hard work. Exercise was a foreign concept because staying alive required moving, hunting, fishing, foraging, and avoiding danger ten to fifteen hours a day. Those who were not agile simply wouldn't survive. The best of the best of us survived and passed those traits down to our children.
- It's been several days with very little food. The dried meat ran out three days ago. Driven by a deep hunger, you search frantically for food. Along the way you find a few berries in the melting spring snow, but they don't do much for that gnawing sensation in the pit of your stomach.
- Up ahead, you hear the hunters shouting with excitement as they corner a young deer. With skill in throwing primitive spears and rocks, a little luck, and a powerful desire to survive, they bring the deer down to the ground. Everyone cheers because tonight, you will have food! It also means you can rest tomorrow because you don't have to hunt. You can set up a base camp and dry and tan the deer's hide, dry pieces of the meat, and take stock of how you're doing. That's a good thing, because you probably took 50,000 steps today.
- Think of how you'll eat the deer meat. Will you eat it slowly, savoring each bite? Or will you gobble it down? Because you're starving and because if you don't, someone else will, you'll eat it as quickly as you can.

Fast forward a couple of hundred thousand years:
- You now have a small farm and some animals fenced in.
- You don't have to get up every day and go out searching for food.

- With all this additional time, you can improve your tools, create art and music, and, unfortunately, invent ways to take over other tribes.
- Still, you end up spending many hours a day doing physical labor and grappling with the inevitable famines that occur about every two years. You average 30,000 steps every day.

Fast forward to today:

- You check your phone for emails and messages.
- You drive to work.
- You sit at a desk and talk to people on the phone, or sit in meetings.
- You pick up lunch at a drive-thru and gobble it down while reading the news and watching clips of late night hosts blasting politicians on your phone.
- You return to work.
- You drive home.
- You eat dinner, read, and watch television—choosing from hundreds of channels and movie/show options.
- Your phone app pedometer registers only 4,500 steps today—about average for Americans.

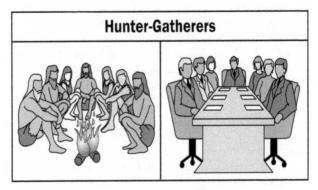

Hunter-Gatherers

You probably understand the huge problem we all face: Our bodies still "think" we are all hunter-gatherers, storing fat efficiently and resisting weight loss aggressively to safeguard against famines of short and long duration. Also, our bodies were designed to move—to move a lot— for most of the day. In the few remaining countries and cultures where people still move a great deal throughout the day, weight problems remain relatively rare. By contrast, modern American culture encourages very sedentary living. A majority of American adults are now overweight at least in part because they don't move enough. Finally, the same biological forces that caused you to quickly gobble up the deer meat are also creating the impulse to gulp down lunch at the drive-through.

It's a wonder everyone isn't overweight. Why do some people remain thin despite these powerful forces?

You undoubtedly know people who seem to eat anything and everything, probably far more than you do, yet remain thin. Our sedentary culture and abundance of foods affects some people far more than others. As you'll see in the remainder of this chapter, some people inherit the tendency to gain weight easily, whereas some inherit the tendency to stay slim. Others who gain weight in middle age, unfortunately, develop those biological tendencies to promote weight gain and resist weight loss later in life. These biological factors have a pronounced impact on weight.

Biological Barriers to Weight Loss

Let's consider some of the details of these biological barriers to help you appreciate and accept their power. Just remember one critical caveat as you read about them:

BIOLOGY IS NOT DESTINY

If biology were fully and completely in charge, no one would ever lose weight and keep it off. Biology makes it tough for athletes to develop the speed, strength, and skills they strive to achieve. Athletes learn how to manage those biological resistances, so do successful weight controllers.

There are actually twelve distinct biological factors that make weight control quite difficult. Whenever people develop excess weight (at any point in their lives), their bodies become especially efficient and effective at maintaining higher-than-normal levels of fat. These biological forces include ones that begin their work before a baby takes its first breath and others that develop over the years. Five of these biological factors are especially impressive and memorable—and may help remind you of the power of this biological foe.

1. **GENES.** Genetic factors are those that are inherited from our parents and prior generations. In breeding studies with mice, fatter mice have been mated with other fatter mice and leaner mice with other leaner mice. Over fifteen to twenty-five generations, this can produce mice pups from the fatter matings with twice as much fat as the pups from the leaner matings. This research shows the tremendous degree to which inheritance of genetic makeup determines the tendency to develop excess fat.

   Human parallels include research showing that children born to parents who are both obese are four times more likely to become obese than children born to lean parents. Some recent research on twins also emphasizes the degree to which inheritance plays a role in developing excess weight. Recall the study by Dr. Bouchard of Canada involving overfeeding twelve pairs of identical twins for one hundred days. If one member of a twin pair gained a lot of weight, the other member of the pair did also. In addition, the twins who gained more weight tended to gain more of the weight as fat and less of it as lean body tissues (such as muscles or organs). Other studies with twins growing up in separate households have shown similar trends: they resembled each other in weight status much more than the siblings with whom they grew up. These findings make it clear that some of us are born with bodies primed to gain weight easily from day one, while others may resist weight gain. Just as genetics dramatically affect weight gain, it similarly affects weight regain after losing it.

2. <u>FAT CELLS = HUNGRY BABY SPARROWS.</u> Beyond genetics, overweight people have more fat cells than people who have never been overweight. How many more? Overweight people can have *four times* as many of these hungry creatures (e.g., 120 billion versus thirty billion). Your fat cells act like hungry baby sparrows, with their mouths wide open looking for more food. Unfortunately, liposuction can only remove a few million of these—barely making a dent because fat is intertwined in our muscles and organs. You can also develop more fat cells at any point in your life. And it doesn't take long to add fat cells. Some studies have shown that animals that are fed large amounts of high-fat food can permanently gain excess fat cells within one week.

Most critically, once fat cells develop, they never disappear. Why is this so important? The importance comes from the fact that fat cells promote very efficient storage of excess food as fat. Studies have traced where the body sends fat after eating. Apparently, for overweight and formerly overweight people, the body delivers fat into the fat cells more efficiently (perhaps directed by some of the biological devices described below). People who have never had weight problems seem to have more fat transported into muscles for use as more immediate fuel.

3. **HORMONES AND ENZYMES.** There are a number of hormones and enzymes that evolution has established as biological barriers to weight loss. While it's not essential that you understand the mechanics of each one, the overall picture is daunting. We'll walk through them one by one to give you a sense of what you're up against.

Insulin. The concentration of blood sugar (glucose) in our bodies is regulated very carefully in people who are not diabetic. The body must maintain this regulation because the brain depends totally on blood sugar for its nutrition. And if our brains aren't properly nourished, we can't survive. This regulation is keyed by a detector in the brain that determines when blood sugar levels are too high or too low. Insulin, which is stored and manufactured in special cells within the pancreas, promotes the ingestion of glucose by our cells.

When people lose weight, the body's fat cells become especially sensitive to insulin. That enables the cells to absorb more nutrients at a faster pace. The muscle cells decrease their sensitivity to insulin, resulting in redirection of fat to the fat cells. Several studies have shown that some people develop an especially high level of insulin sensitivity when they lose weight; these people tend to regain weight very readily. It seems that a great many overweight people are quite sensitive to insulin and can very quickly store excess nutrients as fat, partly because of this tendency. Most overweight people also have excessive amounts of insulin in their blood streams at all times, which may contribute to the efficiency with which their bodies become sensitive to insulin as they lose weight.

LPL. Lipoprotein lipase (LPL) is an enzyme (special

chemical agent) produced in many cells. It stays on the walls of very small blood vessels and can become activated to transport fat in the body. During weight loss, increases in LPL occur as fat cells release their LPL into the bloodstream. By doing so, the fat cells send messages to the brain: "Get more food in us, now!"

Perhaps part of this drive to eat came from attempts to decrease eating occasionally. Biologically, this means that weight loss stimulated hunger and helped convert food into stored fat. At least for some people, LPL activity is especially high and probably makes it more difficult for them to maintain weight loss.

Leptin. Leptin, a hormone discovered in 1994, is secreted by fat cells to act as a messenger between the cells and the brain, directing the amount of fat that gets stored in fat cells by affecting appetite. As fat cells expand during weight gain, leptin is released by those cells. Increasing circulating levels of leptin can decrease appetite and in turn contribute to maintenance of healthy weights; conversely, problems with recognition of leptin in the brain (receptors in the hypothalamus) may increase excess weight.

Ghrelin. The hormone ghrelin is one of the strongest appetite stimulants known. It is produced in the stomach, which releases more ghrelin as people lose weight. For example, one study found that when weight controllers lost seventeen percent of their body weight, their levels of ghrelin rose by twenty-four percent. Further substantiating the importance of ghrelin, weight loss surgery (such as the gastric bypass) decreases ghrelin substantially. With less appetite (due to decreased ghrelin), those who undergo these surgeries don't have to fight the ghrelin battle.

Adiponectin. Adiponectin is a protein secreted by fat cells (like leptin) that helps insulin direct blood sugar from the blood stream into your body's cells. When blood sugar goes into your cells, it is stored or burned for fuel in those cells. Unfortunately, the more fat cells and the larger fat cells a person has, the less adiponectin the fat cells secrete. This effect of adiponectin means that overweight people have a greater propensity to direct blood sugar into fat cells rather than using it for energy.

Between adiponectin, ghrelin, leptin, LPL, and insulin, you can see that the body powerfully resists weight loss for overweight people.

4. **ADAPTIVE THERMOGENESIS.** When weight controllers attempt to lose weight, and reduce the amount of food they consume, their bodies have the capability to switch into a very efficient mode. Remember the plight of the hunter-gatherers, whose bodies we have inherited. In order for them to survive, their bodies had to make adjustments when they couldn't catch a deer in a particular week. Adaptive thermogenesis allowed their bodies to survive on fewer calories (greater efficiency, slower metabolism) during times when adequate amounts of food simply weren't available.

This means that reducing calorie intake by, say, five hundred calories a day may not promote any weight loss if the weight controller's body uses adaptive thermogenesis to switch from its normal mode to a more efficient mode. The good news about adaptive thermogenesis is that you can reverse this effect by moving more than usual or exercising every day. This exercise effect makes it possible for weight controllers to lose weight by bypassing the effects of adaptive thermogenesis (remaining in the relatively inefficient mode that burns more calories).

5. **SET-POINT.** As a weight controller tries to lose weight, his or her body uses adaptive thermogenesis to become efficient. The body also relies on its use of various hormones and enzymes (insulin, leptin, LPL), to make

it difficult to lose weight and keep it off. Fat cells themselves, including their unusual ability to expand in size and number, also contribute to this problem. The set-point concept summarizes all of these effects, making it clear that weight controllers are stuck in bodies that utilize a variety of biological forces to resist weight loss. Just as leptin has been a recent discovery, undoubtedly there are other biological mechanisms that contribute to the body's desire to maintain an excessive amount of fat. Research with animals has shown that very overweight rats and mice show similar tendencies to "defend" (or "set") the amount of fat in their bodies at a high level.

Unfortunately, part of this defense (or set-point) includes a tendency for the bodies of overweight people to respond more dramatically to the sight, smell, and even the thought of tempting foods. A study by psychologists William Johnson and Hal Wildman at the University of Mississippi Medical School confirmed this. These researchers showed that overweight participants, compared to their lean counterparts, increased their insulin responses not only to the actual sight and smell of bacon and eggs, but to the thought of bacon and eggs. The overweight participants also salivated more when they saw or thought about tasty foods. This means that overweight people may defend their high weights by over-secreting insulin and digestive enzymes. These biological responses can increase the desire to consume more food in order to decrease the levels of these substances in the bloodstream.

Accepting the Biological Reality

Now, can you accept the fact that these biological factors create real and powerful resistance to weight loss for you? It's not simply a question of willpower. You face definite biological challenges that require minimizing and managing. There is no escaping this reality. When you think about it, the biology of obesity makes a lot of sense. Why would so many people have so much difficulty maintaining weight losses if biological forces did not resist weight loss? Losing weight produces many positive rewards, but relatively brief lapses in concentration (for example, occasional overeating of high-fat foods and inconsistent exercising) are eagerly greeted by your body's extra billions of fat cells. That's a lot of hungry sparrows to feed! These fat cells and other biological forces are always present, ready to pounce.

The good news here is that once you accept the powerful role that biology plays in creating and maintaining weight problems, you can deflect some of the blame and shame away from your personality or basic self. Weight control is not a question of changing from an abnormal state of gluttony to a normal state of controlled eating. That would be much easier. You must change from a relatively normal state of functioning with an unfortunate biology to a set of behaviors that must be considered super-normal (i.e., beyond the norm, or extraordinary). This makes weight control one of the most difficult challenges a person can face.

Just remember the caveat mentioned earlier in this chapter: **Biology is not destiny.**

Athletes overcome the resistance of their bodies, and so do successful weight controllers.

PSYCHOLOGY. Conscientiousness can help weight controllers and, conversely, emotional instability can interfere with success.

FAMILY. Families that support their weight controllers also can help weight controllers succeed. If families become more active and embrace a very low-fat approach to eating, for example, research shows that their overweight young people succeed at much higher rates than those with less involved families.

<u>EDUCATION.</u> Finally, most people benefit from education about weight control, knowing what to do and how to do it. That includes recipes, and also relevant information about diet and activities. "Knowledge is power" works the other way too. Without knowing the best approach, many weight controllers become influenced by aggressive marketing to believe that some products can help them, when they can't.

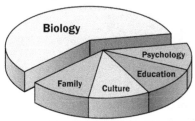

FIGURE 4-4. FIVE CAUSES OF OBESITY.

FIXES

Knowing the causes of weight problems provides some strong suggestions about likely fixes. If a proposed approach ignores the biology of weight management, then it may not help you manage that key aspect of the challenge. Understanding the obesogenic culture, and the insanity of it, can prepare you for the battles ahead as well. The five causes shown in Figure 4-4 suggest that approaches to losing weight and keeping it off really must prepare weight controllers in comprehensive ways. All of the influences can make success either harder or easier, depending on the approach.

Dr. Kristen Gierut (now Kristen Caraher) and I published a paper in which we reviewed five sets of recommendations published by groups of experts on how to help overweight children and teenagers lose weight. The types of treatments that the expert groups considered for young people can be applied to people of all ages. Figure 4-5 illustrates the major options.

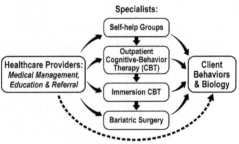

FIGURE 4-5. TREATMENT OPTIONS FOR WEIGHT
MANAGEMENT AND THE PROCESS FLOWING FROM
HEALTHCARE PROVIDERS TO SPECIALISTS TO CLIENTS.

The box on the left side of Figure 4-5 indicates that healthcare providers can help their patients via medical management and offering basic information of relevance to weight controllers. Medical management includes assessment of weight status and potential common complications associated with excess weight, such as high blood pressure, high cholesterol levels, and diabetes. Healthcare providers can also suggest scientifically based books and other materials, as well as make referrals to local specialists. Note the dashed line between the healthcare provider box and actual client behaviors/biology. This means that such medical management and educational information per se rarely produces changes in weight status or lifestyle behaviors. Referrals to specialists, however, can lead to major changes, as indicated by the solid lines between types of specialized interventions and changes in biology and behaviors.

Let's consider in more detail the five primary fixes for weight problems, starting with education. You may notice that I did not include medications in this list of potential fixes. The evidence just does not support the value of current medication for helping overweight people lose substantial amounts of weight in the long run. For example, Orlistat, an FDA approved medication, extracts fat from the food that people eat, essentially helping them consume less fat. But that extracted fat causes many very unpleasant side effects, including uncontrollable bowel movements (not a good thing!). Also, it seems better to follow a very low-fat diet instead of using this medication to produce a similar effect so unnaturally. Chapter 6 explains how to do this most comfortably.

Education

The dashed arrow from the healthcare provider box in Figure 1 to client behaviors suggests that education per se usually fails to help people lose weight. Just telling people what to do simply does not help them do it very well. For example, Dr. Eric Stice and his colleagues provided the first comprehensive review of the effects of educational interventions designed to decrease Body Mass Indexes (BMI, a measure of weight divided by height) in young people. Although most of the sixty-four programs reviewed lasted six months or longer, only twenty-one percent produced statistically reliable reductions in BMI. The reviewers described the average effects of these programs as so small that it "would be considered trivial by most researchers and clinicians." Only three programs—five percent of those evaluated—produced significant effects that persisted over time.

Self-help Groups

Successful weight controllers often report valuing ongoing support to help them succeed. Many studies show beneficial effects from sustained contact, including participation in self-help support groups. These findings support the value of what has been called a "Continuing Care Model" for the treatment of the chronic disease of obesity. For example, a randomized trial of the most widely used approach to self-help groups (Weight Watchers), found that on average, participants in Weight Watchers lost just over three percent of their initial weight. Even this modest average weight loss was substantially better than those who received similar information but didn't attend groups (no sustained weight reduction on average).

Outpatient Cognitive-Behavior Therapy (CBT)

Outpatient CBT programs help people stay focused by encouraging self-monitoring, the writing down of details such as number of fat grams consumed every day. These programs also involve weekly goal setting, planning, problem solving, and mastering stress management skills. Many studies show that people do lose meaningful amounts of weight in such programs and keep the weight off in many cases for years. However, this doesn't happen for most participants, especially those who don't stay involved for at least several months.

Factors that contribute to the variability in outcomes in outpatient CBT approaches include the practical challenges involved with just showing up every week. It's hard to make time in a busy life to go to a meeting, usually in the evenings, every single week. Also, weight loss varies a lot in such programs. During some weeks people gain weight; in other weeks they lose. In a recent paper, Dr. Joseph Skelton and his colleagues reviewed rates of attrition in such outpatient CBT clinics. These authors reported an average attrition of fifty-four percent across five large-scale clinics, including their own. That means more than half of the people who started out in these programs dropped out after only a few weeks. That doesn't provide continuing care at all, regardless of the quality of the programs.

Immersion CBT

Immersion treatment places overweight people in a therapeutic and educational environment for extended periods of time, thereby removing them from obesogenic environments. In contrast to outpatient treatment, immersion treatments, those involving at least ten consecutive days and nights of participation, are more easily accessed by people from diverse locations. Immersion also minimizes the attrition problem that clearly limits the potential impact of outpatient treatment. Immersion treatments for young people and adults have produced promising results. (However, for adults, such programs exist almost exclusively at very expensive health spas.)

Psychologist Kristina Pecora Kelly and I provided the very first comprehensive review of this research, involving twenty-two outcome studies. We concluded that "compared to results highlighted in a recent meta-analysis of outpatient treatments, these immersion programs produced an average of 197 percent greater reductions in percent-overweight at post-treatment and 130 percent greater reduction at follow-up. Furthermore, mean attrition rates were much lower when compared to standard outpatient treatment. Inclusion of a cognitive-behavior therapy (CBT) component seems especially promising; follow-up evaluations showed decreased percent overweight at follow-up by an average of thirty percent for CBT immersion programs versus nine percent for programs without CBT."

I first proposed the Immersion-to-Lifestyle Change model as an explanation for the seemingly promising results obtained in CBT immersion treatments. As shown in Figure 4-6, this model suggests that rapid weight loss combined with CBT may help weight controllers attribute their successes to their own efforts. This, in turn, could increase self-efficacy (self-confidence), reinforce skills like goal setting and self-monitoring, and maximize commitment. The culmination of these effects, in combination with social support, might enhance healthy obsessions. You will read much more about healthy obsessions in the next chapter, Chapter 5, but for now here's my definition (first published in a 2007 book I co-authored, *The Sierras Weight-Loss Solution for Teens and Kids,* and in my 2014 book, *Athlete, Not Food Addict*):

A healthy obsession is a sustained preoccupation with the planning and execution of target behaviors to reach a healthy goal.

This type of intensive focusing definitely seems necessary for success in weight control.

Immersion-to-Lifestyle Change Model

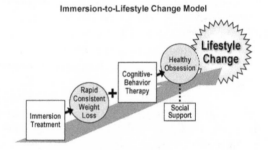

FIGURE 4-6. THE IMMERSION-TO-LIFESTYLE CHANGE MODEL.
REPRINTED WITH PERMISSION FROM MARY ANN LIEBERT, INC.
PUBLISHER: KIRSCHENBAUM, D.S (2010). WEIGHT LOSS CAMPS IN THE US
AND THE IMMERSION-TO-LIFESTYLE CHANGE MODEL. *CHILDHOOD OBESITY, 6, 318-323.*

Bariatric Surgery

Bariatric surgery holds some promise, but this extreme intervention quite often creates troublesome side effects and is only available for limited numbers of extremely overweight people. Many very overweight people do benefit from this rather major procedure, but most overweight and obese people would find their lives disrupted less by using the present approach to succeed instead.

SUMMARY

Table 4-1 summarizes the effects of the five approaches to fix weight problems considered in this chapter. As you can see, education rarely seems to produce benefits in the long run by itself. In combination with outpatient CBT or self-help, quite a few people can improve their health and happiness grounded in useful knowledge. Bariatric surgery may produce more substantial improvements for extremely overweight people, but it often comes with significant financial and physical costs. Finally, immersion CBT seems quite promising for those who can afford such programs.

For those who cannot afford the more expensive approaches, good self-help programs may prove quite useful. These come closest to providing the continuing care focus that many people find helpful. For all weight controllers, obtaining a thorough knowledge of what helps (i.e., using TUS) and what doesn't provides the foundation for change. By reviewing the next four chapters describing the remaining four steps of the present approach, you can refine your understanding of what it takes to succeed as a weight controller-athlete.

EFFECTIVENESS OF FIVE APPROACHES TO WEIGHT MANAGEMENT	
Education	• Minimal effects • 5% may benefit significantly
Self-Help	• 10-33% may benefit long-term.
Outpatient Cognitive-Behavior Therapy	• 20-50% may benefit long-term.
Bariatric Surgery	• 33-50% substantial improvement, but available for limited population. • Some post-surgical complications.
Immersion CBT Programs	• Good potential for long-term change • Perhaps 33-50% benefit long term.

TABLE 4-1

CHAPTER 5
Losing Weight Permanently

HOP STEP 2: DEVELOPING A HEALTHY OBSESSION

Persistence

Nothing in the world can take the place of persistence.
Talent will not;
Nothing is more common than unsuccessful people
  with talent.
Genius will not;
Unrewarded genius is almost a proverb.
Education will not;
The world is full of educated derelicts.
Persistence and determination alone are omnipotent.

–CALVIN COOLIDGE, 1932

This perspective by President Coolidge hits upon a concept that rings true for every coach, every graduate admissions committee, and most employers. These decision-makers all seek candidates who persist in the face of challenges. They aim to populate their teams, programs, and companies with people who persist despite inevitable obstacles, almost regardless of innate talent.

Basketball great Ernie DiGregorio understood this when he was twelve years old:

"Nobody gets up at six in the morning to play ball, but I did. At twelve years old, my mind was made up: I was going to play pro ball ... I started practicing nine, ten hours

a day by myself, with gloves, and I loved it. They could've cut my right hand off and I'd have played one-handed."

The "Great One," Wayne Gretzky, was renowned for his work ethic on and off the ice. Wayne believes that *"The highest compliment that you can pay me is to say that I worked hard every day, that I never dogged it."*

Most people know this innately: persistence wins in the end. But the question remains: "How can I create this in myself or nurture it?" This is exactly the purpose of the overarching mission in the approach used in this book: to develop a healthy obsession.

THE HEALTHY OBSESSION

Although the word obsession tends to have negative connotations in the outside world, in the present approach I use the word "obsession" to refer to persistent thoughts that compel actions. If an obsession is healthy, it will help you achieve a positive way of living. For weight controllers, a healthy obsession is a very strong drive toward achieving the three primary goals of this approach: eating very little fat, getting 12,000 steps per day, and self-monitoring one hundred percent. A healthy obsession results in more daydreams, plans, and routines that help maintain key behaviors. Remember, weight control is an athletic challenge—overcoming a biology that resists achievement of the goal. Also, our obesogenic culture makes it even harder to succeed. It's like trying to run a five-minute mile into a strong headwind. Our biology and the headwind won't give us a break, nor do they give partial credit for moderate, albeit sincere, efforts.

It requires a great deal of persistence to become a successful weight controller. That's the healthy obsession, focusing the weight controller on consistency of eating, moving, and self-monitoring—to overcome these barriers to success.

DEFINITION

A healthy obsession is a sustained preoccupation with the planning and execution of target behaviors to reach a healthy goal. You may recall this definition from earlier in this chapter and in a prior chapter, but I first described this phrase in my 1994 book, *Weight Loss Through Persistence.* I greatly expanded on it in my 2014 book, *Athlete, Not Food Addict.* Some other elements of the definition include:

A healthy obsession is:

- Knowing that your biology has turned against you and does not go on vacations or cut you slack because "you've had a rough day."
- Accepting the tough goal of eating as little fat as possible every day.
- Knowing that "the devil is in the details" so that writing down all food eaten is critical.
- Understanding that everything counts—everything.
- Being very reluctant to accept permission, even from yourself, to overindulge.
- Making plans to help yourself stick with this program at parties, at restaurants, and on trips.
- Analyzing lapses in order to prevent the same problem from happening tomorrow.
- Refusing to allow lapses to become relapses.
- Refusing to let a number on a scale prevent you from persisting.
- Feeling anxious if the goals in this program are not met.
- Accepting the idea that activity every day is the way, and doing it—even when you don't feel like it.
- Being an active problem solver, oriented to take action, not just to analyze.

A healthy obsession is NOT:
- Seeking moderation in all things.
- Giving yourself permission to deviate from the program because of moods, stress, holidays, or vacations.
- Waltzing into a high-risk situation (like a party or a Mexican restaurant) without a plan.
- Making lame excuses for major lapses.
- Allowing lapses to turn into relapses.
- Feeling just fine when goals are sometimes not met.
- Getting thrown into a major tailspin because a number on a scale is too high.
- Wallowing in self-pity.
- Getting discouraged and overwhelmed.

A HEALTHY OBSESSION STARTS WITH SELF-MONITORING

Every diet requires some change in eating patterns and a reduction in calories consumed. But diets also give weight controllers hope and—even more importantly—increase awareness. The most helpful aspects of any diet lie in these factors, not in the magic of grapefruit or the latest ideas in combining foods. Self-monitoring can create that awareness better than any other behavioral strategy.

The key behavioral component for successful long-term weight control is self-monitoring, the systematic observation of key behaviors (eating and moving), and the recording of those observations.

"A person who wishes to change himself should demand an account of himself with regard to the particular point which he has resolved to watch in order to correct himself and improve. Let him go over the single hours or periods from the time he arose to the hour and moment

of the present examination and make a mark for each time he has fallen into the particular sin or defect. The second day should be compared with the first, that is, the two examinations of the present day with the two of the preceding day. Let him observe if there is an improvement from one day to another. Let him compare one week with another and observe whether he has improved during the present week as compared to the preceding."
                                    —St. Ignatius Loyola, 1500

St. Ignatius Loyola's thoughts on behavioral change date from the Middle Ages, but they remain remarkably accurate today based on current scientific knowledge. Researchers have demonstrated the importance of self-monitoring to improve performance across a wide range of disciplines. Self-monitoring is used extensively in sports. Professional football players want to know how fast they run the forty-yard dash. Pitchers want to know how fast and how accurately they are pitching. Feedback is the key ingredient for improved performance. In one famous study, Olympic-level figure skaters were left to train on their own. They attempted sixty elements (jumps, spins) in an hour of training. Then a whiteboard was brought out onto the ice so their coach could tally the number of jumps and spins in real time. The result: the number of elements attempted rose from sixty to one hundred. Then the whiteboard was removed, and the number declined to sixty. Then the coach brought the whiteboard out again. The result: suddenly the figure skaters were attempting one hundred elements again.

Many scientific studies have demonstrated the importance of self-monitoring for successful long-term weight control. Simply put, weight controllers who self-monitor consistently lose much more weight and keep if off much better than those who don't self-monitor consistently. Leading obesity researcher, Dr. Tom Wadden of the University of Pennsylvania, in 1993 described self-monitoring as the "cornerstone" of behavioral treatment for weight problems.

What is Self-Monitoring? Thousands of participants in my programs, including Wellspring, used the two pages below in a sixty-page booklet called self-monitoring journals or SMJs:

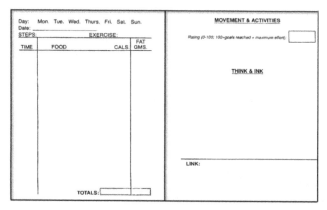

Here's how participants using the program described in this book use their SMJs: At the beginning of each day, they circle the day of the week and write down the date. Then, at breakfast, they write down everything they ate. This includes:

- What you're eating,
- Portion size (# of ounces or cups),
- Calories,
- Fat grams.

They repeat the process for lunch, dinner, and snacks. They're advised to write down something—anything—that occurs to them in the "Think & Ink" section. This section comprises a journaling technique. Journaling, just writing down thoughts and feelings without focusing on the quality of the writing, can improve focus, management of moods, and promote success in various tasks. The "Link" section allows the weight controller to extract key thoughts or ideas about the day.

At the end of the day, participants in these programs:

- Recorded steps where it says STEPS (top left).
- Totaled their calories and fat grams for the day.
- Reviewed how active they were—on a scale of one to one hundred with one hundred being as active as you possibly could be; was today a twenty or an eighty (top right of the second page)?

You may be wondering: "How will I know how many calories or fat grams are in a particular food?" Many weight controllers use a wonderful pocket-sized booklet mentioned in the food chapter called *CalorieKing— Calorie, Fat & Carbohydrate Counter* (written by dietitian Allan Borushek and updated annually). This book is also available online (www.calorieking.com) and as an app for smart phones, as are other calorie and fat counters.

Why is Self-Monitoring So Important? Self-monitoring helps people maximize their commitment to their goals, stay committed to them, feel in control, understand their patterns of eating and moving, focus on the details, and even keep their moods more positive. The box below provides another summary of these points.

Why Self-Monitoring Helps

Consistent self-monitoring improves weight control by:

- Increasing ability to use GOALS
- Improving COMMITMENT to change
- Increasing coping and feelings of CONTROL
- Improving understanding of EATING/ EXERCISE PATTERNS
- Improving information about, and focus on, the DETAILS
- Promoting more POSITIVE MOODS

The experiences of participants in these programs strongly suggest the power of self-monitoring. Decades of scientific research confirm its importance.

Science Supports the Value of Self-monitoring. No researcher or health care professional who is familiar with the scientific literature on weight control would disagree with the value of self-monitoring. Table 5-1 shows some of the findings from studies on this very point. The results demonstrate that *when people write down at least seventy-five percent of their eating and exercising behaviors, they are much more likely to be successful in losing weight and maintaining weight loss. Failing to write down these critical aspects of weight control tends to result in minimal or temporary success.*

RESEARCH ON THE BENEFITS OF VERY CONSISTENT SELF-MONITORING

Weight controllers who discontinued self-monitoring during the holiday season (Thanksgiving to New Year's) gained fifty-seven times more weight than their counterparts who continued to self-monitor consistently.

Two studies showed that even weight controllers who self-monitor very consistently often discontinue monitoring for a day or more. During the weeks when they took a day or more "off," they lost much less weight than usual. Specifically, when these consistent self-monitors kept track of virtually everything they ate and all of their activity, they lost between one and two pounds per week. In contrast, during their least consistent weeks, they lost only half as much weight.

Weight controllers who were generally inconsistent self-monitors gained an average of one pound per week during their least consistent self-monitoring weeks. They fared much better—in fact they maintained their weight—during weeks in which they self-monitored almost every day.

In two different studies, only highly consistent self-monitors lost any weight during the holiday season (Thanksgiving to New Year's); see the featured research presented on the next page.

Weight controllers who self-monitored very consistently in the first few weeks of several outpatient professional treatment programs maintained much greater weight losses, compared to inconsistent self-monitors, when evaluated one to two years after treatment began.

In two follow-up studies conducted one to one and a half years after participants completed their stays in one of the Wellspring camps, results showed that highly successful campers used self-monitoring after camp far more often than unsuccessful campers.

TABLE 5-1

FEATURED RESEARCH: SELF-MONITORING CONSISTENTLY PRODUCES CONSISTENTLY SUPERIOR RESULTS

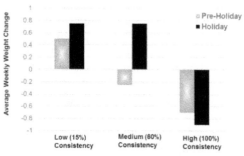

Based on Baker, R. C. & Kirschenbaum, D. S. (1998). Weight control during the holidays: The potentially critical role of self-monitoring. *Health Psychology, 17,* 367-379.

The author and Dr. Ray Baker recorded the consistency of self-monitoring by thirty-eight well-educated participants (fifty-eight percent had completed college) in a cognitive-behavior therapy (CBT) program for weight control. Consistency rates (varying from zero percent, meaning not recording anything for the prior two weeks, to one hundred percent) determined which of the categories into which each participant belonged (Low, Medium, or High Consistency), as shown in the figure above. Those in the Low Consistency group averaged about one to two days per week of self-monitoring, whereas those in High Consistency group recorded something every day.

As the figure shows, Low Consistency participants gained weight during the holiday weeks (Thanksgiving and Christmas weeks) and non-holiday weeks (the weeks right before the holidays). The Medium group gained almost one pound during the holiday weeks on average, but lost weight in the non-holiday weeks. Only the High Consistency group (one hundred percent self-monitoring), lost weight even during the high-risk holiday weeks. So, based on this study (and several others), it appears that consistent self-monitoring can protect weight controllers from re-gaining weight even during times of high risk, like the holidays with all of the parties, big meals, and abundant high-fat foods.

Does it Matter How You Monitor? Possibly. Many weight controllers use online programs or phone apps. The research indicates that consistency matters a lot, but it remains unclear if the format of self-monitoring matters. In my experience with hundreds of clients in recent years, it seems that self-monitoring the old-fashioned way, in writing, has an advantage over using apps or other electronic monitoring. Just seeing the details in writing every day may improve focus and commitment more effectively. Also, it's an easier process, less impacted by confusing rules that affect electronic systems. When you write down a chicken sandwich, you can just write down "chicken sandwich" and note the three fat grams and 320 calories. Using an app may require looking up the bread, the chicken, and other aspects of the sandwich—much more work.

Bottom line: this very simple saying can help summarize the healthy obsession that self-monitoring helps promote:

Everything Counts!

Weight control does not begin on a Monday or on the first day of a new month or on the first day of a new year. It begins as soon as weight controllers make a sincere effort to control eating and increase moving. By making everything count, self-monitoring helps create the foundation to the broader concept, the key attitude and approach, defined by the term "healthy obsession."

Science of Healthy Obsession

Decades of research strongly suggest the benefits of a healthy obsession for successful long-term weight control. The following summarize some of the more compelling findings:

- Perhaps the most consistent finding over the past thirty years in the weight-loss literature is that when weight controllers regularly attend professionally conducted weight-loss therapy, they usually persist and succeed at losing weight almost every week.

Two studies randomly assigned people to groups in which they received either long-term or short-term professional behavioral weight-loss therapy. In both studies, the groups that received a longer course of treatment lost far more weight. Attending weekly sessions helps people focus on the details of their eating, greatly increases their consistency of self-monitoring, and promotes the development of a healthy obsession (e.g., more planning and problem solving).

- In a series of studies, psychologist Michael Perri and his colleagues from the University of Florida found that almost any effort that consistently focused the attention of their clients on the process of losing weight improved maintenance of weight loss. Comparing different types of booster sessions held weekly over six months, the researchers found that sessions focused on relapse prevention or problem solving did not help maintain weight losses any better than those focused on very general discussions of recipes and other weight-loss issues. The conclusion: Any kind of contact—even sending postcards or making brief phone calls, regardless of the content—improved the ability of weight controllers to maintain weight loss as compared to people who did not receive such attention. Attention from concerned others leads to more intensive focus on goals, plans, and commitments (i.e., healthy obsessions).

- The National Weight Control Registry includes responses to surveys by more than two thousand people who have lost, on average, fifty pounds and kept it off for six years. On average, these master weight controllers (Long-Term Weight Controllers or LTWCs) lost and regained 270 pounds before they were finally successful. Another survey of two hundred LTWCs found that final success came only after an average of five previous temporarily successful weight losses. The reason they finally succeeded? A much more intensive approach. In fact, the majority of LTWCs in the National Weight Control Registry used a much stricter dietary regimen (very low-fat) and more than eighty percent reported they exercised far more than in previous attempts. They also reported paying much more careful attention to their weight, their eating, and their activity.

- Another study by Dr. Michael Perri and his colleagues focused on 379 sedentary adults who wanted to become more active and fit. Half of the participants were asked to walk for thirty minutes three to four days per week (moderate approach) while the other half was asked to walk for the same duration five to seven days per week (intensive approach). The researchers expected the moderate approach (goal of three to four walks per week) to result in more walking than the intensive approach (goal of five to seven walks per week) over time. The healthy obsession concept would argue that the researchers expected the wrong results. Daily activity improves focus and should generally lead to more consistent activity over the long haul. Sure enough, over a six-month period, the more intensive approach led to fifty-three percent more walking than the moderate approach.

- A study by psychologist Eric Stice of Stanford University makes a related point about dieting. Dr. Stice followed a large sample of teens ages sixteen to nineteen over nine months. Dr. Stice found that many were dieting to some extent. The most important finding from this study is that moderate levels of dieting were associated with weight *gain* while more intensive forms were associated with weight *loss*. Dr. Stice's intensive dieters, for example, regularly used eighteen out of nineteen possible dietary behaviors in order to try to lose weight. Moderate dieters reported using only half of these dietary behaviors.

• Wellspring researchers conducted two studies involving intensive interviews with either very successful or unsuccessful campers more than a year post-camp. These studies involved asking a series of probing questions about healthy obsessions using the "Wellspring Transformative Change Interview." In one of those studies, Kristen Caraher and I found both numerical (quantitative) and qualitative differences between the successful weight controllers (named "Losers" in this study) and unsuccessful weight controllers ("Gainers"). Here's how we summarized those differences. The numbers in front of the questions in italics indicate the number of the question in the survey (out of fifty-three total questions asked of the participants):

<u>QUANTITATIVE DIFFERENTIATORS.</u> *29. You're on vacation with your family for ten days. On how many of those days would you eat twenty grams of fat or less?* Losers reported they would eat less than twenty grams of fat per day on almost twice as many days on that vacation than Gainers (M = 6.38 vs. 3.44 days).

34-36. You have three major exams coming up in school this week. You have to meet with groups, cram/study very hard, and you feel very stressed about getting everything done and doing well. Of the seven days leading up to the exam, how many days would you monitor food? How many days would you get 10,000 steps? How many days would you eat twenty grams of fat or less? Losers reported they would continue to self-monitor an average of 5.25 days leading up

to the exam vs. 3.94 days by Gainers. Losers indicated they
would exercise on average 4.94 days leading up to the exam
compared to 3.38 days by the Gainers. Losers also reported
they would eat less than twenty grams of fat per day on an
average of 5.88 days leading up to the exam vs. 4.69 days
by Gainers.

39. *You get into a fight with your best friend (boyfriend/
girlfriend), and he/she does not speak to you for the rest
of the day. Will you still eat less than twenty grams of fat
on this day?* All Losers (8/8) reported they would still eat
less than twenty grams of fat on this day whereas only half
of the Gainers (4/8) reported they would still eat less than
twenty grams of fat on this day.

42-43. *You are heading to your friend's house for a
party. You know that the food there will primarily consist
of high-fat pizza and chips. Will you still reach your 10,000-
step goal today? Will you still eat less than twenty grams
of fat this day?* All Losers, eight out of eight, indicated they
would still reach their step goal vs. five out of eight of the
Gainers. Similarly, all Losers (8/8) reported they would still
eat less than twenty grams of fat on this day whereas only
five of the Gainers (5/8) reported they would eat within
that key guideline of the present approach.

QUALITATIVE DIFFERENTIATORS. 26. *Let's
imagine that you normally get in 10,000 steps every day by
walking, but today your ankle really hurts; you injured it
playing soccer yesterday, and it is uncomfortable to walk.
Will this impact the food you eat this day?* Only Losers
demonstrated attitudes consistent with a healthy obsession
by noting that they would decrease their eating because
they expected the injury to prevent them from reaching
their activity goals. In sharp contrast, two of the Gainers
noted that they expected to overeat in response to the
injury, not decrease their eating.

For example, one Loser stated, "Yes it would [impact
the food I eat]. You have to change your diet since you'll

do less exercise. You still need to lose weight that day." Another Loser mentioned, "I would make sure I'm being very careful of what I'm eating because I cannot meet my step goal." In contrast, a Gainer stated, "Probably [impact the food I eat], more in a negative way. I would probably feel sorry for myself. I would be less likely to get up and cook things because my ankle would hurt and go out and get healthy things is unlikely if I'm injured." Another Gainer stated, "Um, I do find myself getting bored in situations like this and then I'd just eat more."

37. *You get into a fight with your best friend (boyfriend/ girlfriend), and he/she does not speak to you for the rest of the day. How does this impact your activity for the day?* Losers again demonstrated more substantial healthy obsessions than Gainers. Losers reported that the fight with their friend would not impact their weight control programs whereas Gainers expected negative outcomes. For example, one Loser stated, "I'll suck it up and do what I need to do. It wouldn't affect me." Similarly, another Loser reported, "It [fight with friend] doesn't impact my activity; well, to me that's a non-related event. You must exercise, and you cannot let things hinder you." In contrast a Gainer stated, "Um, I'd sit there eating frozen yogurt and watch TV and cry. It affects me very much when I get into an argument." Another Gainer mentioned, "lower it [my activity] dramatically."

41. *You are heading to your friend's house for a party. You know that the food there will primarily consist of high-fat pizza and chips. Do you have a plan for eating at the party?* Losers used more definitive language about their plans, whereas Gainers used language such as "probably" and "I guess," illustrating less confidence in their responses. For example, one Loser stated, "Yes [I have a plan]. I'll bring a Lean Cuisine. I don't care what people say."

Another Loser stated, "Yes, I would eat before. It's a little trick that I do, because if you are already full you are not going to eat anything else. And just be like 'oh, no I am not hungry thank you.' I would definitely eat before and make sure that it was fulfilling food so that I am satisfied." In contrast, a Gainer predicted, "Probably eat one plate and a few chips and go hang out."

- Many other studies in peer-reviewed journals support the healthy obsession concept. We know, for example, that weight controllers who have greater stability in their lives because of their jobs, financial situations, and mental health succeed more often than those with unstable personal and work situations. Some studies even find that older adults—those over sixty—tend to succeed more in professional weight loss programs than younger adults. One strong hypothesis is that greater stability in life allows weight controllers to focus more clearly on developing very consistent patterns, a key element in healthy obsessions.

Nurturing a Healthy Obsession

Self-monitoring consistently provides the most direct route to developing a healthy obsession. This chapter documented how powerfully both self-monitoring and healthy obsessions can impact success. The figure below makes the key point about healthy obsessions: It's fundamentally a choice in life. You either go down the road toward this challenging but rewarding way of living or you stay on the other side of it (and therefore fail to achieve your weight loss goals). Just as serious athletes must make substantial commitments to their sport every day, so do weight controllers. *You cannot dangle your big toe in this process and expect to succeed.*

Make Your Choice - Don't Look Back

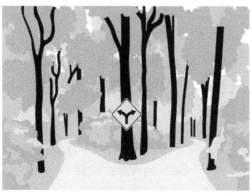

Another direction for nurturing your own healthy obsession comes from those around you and the environments in which you live and work every day. Very few athletes excel on their own, without encouragement and support around them. The final chapter (Step 5 of HOP) focuses on how to build that winning team for your weight controlling efforts.

CHAPTER 6
Losing Weight Permanently

HOP STEP 3: EATING TO LOSE—THREE MAJOR DIETARY PRINCIPLES

This chapter can help you tame those extra billions of fat cells, which make their presence known to your appetite every day. Thousands of very successful weight controllers have managed to satisfy these hungry cells; you can too.

In this chapter you will learn that three dietary principles have the greatest impact on your hunger, weight, and long-term prospects for success: very low fat (VLF), low caloric density, and controlled calories. HOP works best when you base your overall style of eating in a healthful, balanced approach to food. The "Healthy Eating Basics" described below can help you develop that solid foundation to your weight controlling efforts.

Healthy Eating Basics: A Balanced Approach

To encourage Americans to eat a varied and balanced diet, and thereby consume adequate amounts of vitamins, minerals, and fiber, the U.S. Department of Agriculture officially launched the Food Guide Pyramid in 1992. In 2011, the USDA replaced the pyramid with the "my plate" icon, pictured below. The USDA plate presents five food groups, with the grain group (bread, cereal, rice, and pasta) and the vegetable group taking up most of the space.

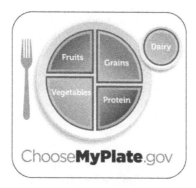

The USDA website, http://myplate.gov/, has tremendous amounts of information, available as videos and posters and tips of the day, among other things. These materials promote a balanced diet that would allow you to get all of the essential nutrients and vitamins. The following descriptions summarize *their* recommendations (not the ideal ones for weight controllers, as you will discover) about the five food groups, with recommended numbers of servings based on a 2,000 calorie per day diet:

<u>Vegetables: 2.5 cups per day</u>
- 1 cup = a cup of raw or cooked vegetables; 2 cups of leafy salad vegetables = 1 cup of cooked vegetables
- Eat more red, orange, and dark-green vegetables
- Add beans or peas to salads, soups, and side dishes
- Fresh, frozen, and canned vegetables all can work.

<u>Fruits: 2 cups per day</u>
- 1 cup = raw, cooked or 100% juice; ½ cup of dried fruit counts the same as 1 cup of raw fruit
- Use fruits as snacks, salads, and desserts
- Top your cereal at breakfast with bananas or berries

<u>Grains: 6 ounces per day</u>
- 1 ounce = 1 slice of bread, ½ cup cooked pasta, rice, or cereal

- Substitute whole-grain choices for refined grains
- Choose products that name a whole grain first on the ingredients list

Dairy: 3 cups per day
- 1 cup = a cup of milk, yogurt, or soymilk; 1.5 ounces of natural cheese
- Choose skim or 1% milk
- Top baked potatoes with low-fat yogurt

Protein Foods: 5.5 ounces per day
- 1 ounce = 1 ounce of lean meat, poultry, or fish; 1 egg; 1 tablespoon peanut butter; .5 oz nuts or seeds; .25 cup of beans or peas
- Eat a variety of foods from this group each week, such as seafood, beans and peas, and nuts, as well as lean meats, poultry, and eggs
- Chose lean meats, trim or drain fat, and have seafood twice a week

If you follow the guidelines provided by My Plate, you probably will not benefit from taking vitamin or mineral supplements of any kind. However, because very few people follow this balanced approach, you may benefit from taking a multi-vitamin once per day. You can also see by the examples that many low-fat, low-calorie foods can be used to create a balanced meal plan. On the other hand, the plan you will find in the remainder of this chapter emphasizes an even lower fat approach to eating.

Having an overall grasp of healthful, balanced eating provides the foundation for using HOP's three keys to eating for weight loss. Please review those keys in Table 6-1 before beginning to read about the first key: very low-fat eating.

VLF HOP's Three Major Dietary Principles
EAT:
1. Very Low Fat (VLF—aim for 0; 20 fat g maximum)
2. Low Caloric-Density (i.e., foods with few calories per gram of weight or ounce of volume)
3. Caloric Control: 1,200-1,800 Calories per Day

TABLE 6-1

GOOD-BYE FAT

"Any pig farmer knows that you can't get pigs fat feeding them wheat; you need corn, which contains more oil," says Professor Elliot Danforth. Danforth and his colleague Ethan Sims, both professors at the University of Vermont, studied the causes of obesity. Using male prisoners as subjects, they asked the prisoners to eat large amounts of food and then observed the effects. They found that the prisoners who ate a lot of high-fat foods gained much more weight than those who ate foods that were lower in fat and higher in carbohydrates.

High-fat foods are most easily stored as additional fat in the body. For example, to turn one hundred calories of very high-fat foods like butter or bacon into body fat, your body only expends about three calories of energy. That means that ninety-seven of the one hundred calories end up in your fat cells. Turning carbohydrates into fat is much more complicated. The body has to change the carbohydrate into a number of other chemical compounds in order to process it. As a result, in order to turn one hundred calories of spaghetti into fat, the body has to expend about twenty-three calories. In other words, it costs very little energy to transform foods that start out as fat into body fat. Therefore, one hundred calories of spaghetti may translate into seventy-seven calories of fat, whereas one hundred calories of butter transform into ninety-seven calories of fat.

You can see from the information already presented that eating foods high in fat can lead to weight gain, in part by the efficiency with which your body stores fat. The previous chapter showed other aspects of your biology that promote weight gain and resist weight loss. In the present dietary approach, very low fat takes center stage—the first and most important element of how to eat to lose weight. Let's consider several other factors/findings that help justify making this key principle top of the list of three dietary recommendations.

Rationale for a Very Low-Fat Diet

I began advocating for a very low-fat diet about two decades ago (e.g., *The 9 Truths about Weight Loss*, published in 2000). A few years after the publication of that popular book, I created the dietary and other aspects of what became the leading provider of treatment services for overweight young people in America, as noted in prior chapters: Wellspring (weight loss camps and boarding schools, starting in 2004). Wellspring's published results rival any weight-loss program ever evaluated, and those results were published in several scientific journals (2004-2014).

In contrast to a very low-fat approach, the low-carb diets focus on nearly eliminating carbohydrates from the diet and replacing many of those calories with fat. Despite its sustained popularity over the decades, no health organization advocates using low-carb diets (e.g., American Heart Association, American Dietetic Association). For example, for the past seven years, *US News and World Report* organized a group of twenty experts to comment on the best diets. They consistently rate diets low or very low in fat at the top of their lists, including the Dietary Approach to Stop Hypertension

(DASH), Dean Ornish's Diet (very low fat), and Weight Watchers (low fat). In another great example, the editor in chief of the top specialty journal focused on this topic, *Obesity*, physician/researcher George Blackburn, wrote an important editorial in 2008, "The Low-Fat Imperative." He argued persuasively that research comparing different diets no longer seemed worthwhile. Instead, "our task is not to debate whether low-fat diets work, but to find ways to increase adherence to them."

These strong opinions favoring low-fat or very low-fat diets come from decades of research on animals and humans. That research keeps making the point that fat increases weight gain and contributes more than any other nutrient to difficulties with losing weight. Fat increases appetite, promotes fat storage, and works against weight loss in many other ways (e.g., promotes weight re-gain among those, both human and animals, who have already lost weight). Furthermore, no other dietary approach has ever shown a benefit comparable to a low-fat or a very low-fat approach, despite what the sellers of snake oil and other fake approaches claim on a daily basis in their articles, blogs, and best-sellers. Table 6-2 summarizes this overwhelming evidence in favor of very low-fat eating plans, as well as mentioning some other documented findings. The two featured research studies below also support this perspective. Convinced yet?

SUMMARY OF BENEFITS OF
VERY LOW-FAT DIETS (VLFS)

Very successful weight controllers use LF or VLF diets almost exclusively.

Dietary instructions alone (without counseling) focused on VLFs promote weight loss more effectively than other instructions (e.g., focused on carbohydrates or total calories).

VLFs promote improved stability of hormones that impact hunger (e.g., Leptin, Grehlin).

LFs improve moods compared to low carbohydrate (LC) diets.

LC (and high-fat) diets did the opposite of what a group of researchers who advocated for an LC approach expected: it slowed loss of fat compared to a higher carbohydrate/lower fat diet of the same number of total calories.

Epidemiological studies of teenagers and adults show that fat consumption, not carbohydrate consumption, predicted weight gain.

Animal studies consistently show that VLF diets decrease appetite, promote weight loss, and decrease weight re-gain more effectively than other diets.

Research on programs and cultures that focus on VLF diets show major benefits for health compared to usual diets.

Expert opinion consistently favors LFs or VLFs, e.g., editor of the major specialty journal in the field, *Obesity*, in 2008 called for a "low-fat imperative"—no longer necessary to debate type of diet, just to figure out how to help people adhere to LFs/VLFs; for the past seven years, *US News & World Report's* twenty dietary experts have consistently favored LFs or VLFs as the dietary approaches that work best.

TABLE 6-2

Featured Research: Very Low-Fat Diet +
Cognitive Behavior Therapy (CBT) Improves Heart Health

Physician/researcher Dean Ornish and his colleagues conducted some of the most important studies in the history of research on heart health. They randomly assigned about thirty people who had painful and dangerous blockages in their coronary arteries (the ones supplying the heart with fresh blood) to a "Treatment" group. That group, pictured below, received twice weekly Cognitive Behavior Therapy (CBT) group sessions, yoga, and meals prepared with very little fat (VLF). Members of that CBT + VLF Treatment group self-monitored their eating and attempted to eat very little fat every day. The other group of about thirty people, the "Usual Care" group, just did the usual things recommended for cardiac patients—went to cardiac rehabilitation programs, saw their cardiologists regularly, and so on.

As you can see below, the Treatment group actually decreased the amount of blockages in their coronary arteries over time, far more so and by using less medicine than the Usual Care group. They also had about half as many subsequent cardiac events, including heart attacks and surgical interventions. The Treatment group also lost significantly more weight and kept it off compared to the Usual Care group.

CBT Support + Very Low Fat Diet: 5 Year Follow-up

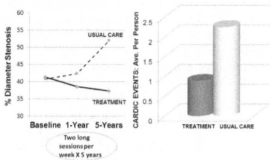

Ornish, D. et al. (1998). Intensive lifestyle changes for reversal of coronary heart disease. *JAMA, 280,* 2001-7.

Featured Research: The Heart Healthiest Population in the World Today—The Tsimane of Bolivia, South America

Anthropologist Hillard Kaplan and twenty of his colleagues from around the world discovered that the Tsimane people eat a low-fat (almost a very low-fat) diet, get more than four times more steps per day than average Americans (17,000 vs. 4,000), and, quite remarkably, have almost no heart disease—even among their older adults. The two figures below show that objectively measured Coronary Artery Disease (CAD) differed dramatically between a very large sample of people in the US (pictured below in different age groupings, 65-74 and 75-84). As you can see, in the US, as people go from the younger of these two age groupings to the more elderly grouping, CAD increases from about thirty to fifty percent. Among the Tsimane, CAD remains for both groupings at about eight percent, radically lower levels. The Tsimane also have much lower rates of obesity and eat a diet that has less than half the fat of the average American diet.

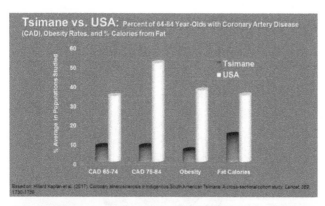

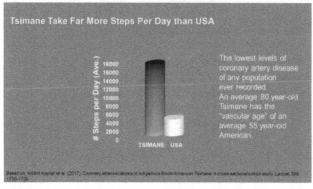

Fat Goal: How Low Can You Go?

Aim for Zero Fat Grams

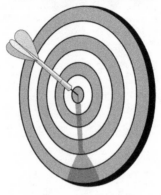

In order to avoid eating fat, it helps to know how to measure the amount of fat in your diet. To do that, it helps to either buy a great calorie and fat gram counter, the best of which is the pocket sized *The CalorieKing Calorie, Fat & Carbohydrate Counter* by Allan Borushek (updated annually). CalorieKing also has a great website and app if you'd prefer a more high-tech approach. Certain types of fat (like saturated fats, trans fats) create more cardiovascular health problems than other types of fat (for example, polyunsaturated fats such as olive oil and monounsaturated fats such as peanut oil). However, successful weight controllers generally in HOP eat so little fat that they don't have to worry much at all about which types of fat they consume. From an HOP weight-control perspective:

A fat is a fat is a fat.

In other words, all fats contain approximately the same number of calories. And, your body stores all fats very readily. In this respect:

1 tablespoon of peanut oil = lard = corn oil
= coconut oil = butter =
120 calories and 13.6 fat grams.

So, the question of greatest concern to those who want to lose weight is, "How little fat can I get myself to eat?"

Some studies indicate that obese people consume higher percentages of their calories from fat than lean people. Most obese people eat similar numbers of total calories compared to non-obese individuals, but the percentages of fat in their diets can be twenty-five percent higher. If you want to lose weight, you must consume very little fat every day. The American Heart Association suggests that if Americans adopted a diet consisting of thirty percent of calories from fat, there would be much less heart disease in this country. Right now, Americans consume closer to thirty-four percent of their total calories from fat. Reducing to diets containing thirty percent fat might improve the health of some people, but this level is still far too high for you and others who wish to lose weight. Some experts recommend that a better percentage for weight controllers is twenty percent. My recommendation is even simpler than that: consume as little fat as possible (and certainly less than ten percent of all calories from fat)—and just add up the total number of fat grams you consume each day, regardless of the percentage of calories from fat. So, the answer to the question, "How low can you go?" is, "As low as possible."

Aim for zero fat grams per day and accept
no more than twenty grams.

Not only is this no-fat goal clearer than ten percent or twenty percent of calories from fat, but research suggests it works better too.

Living with a VLF eating plan presents challenges. This is the age of motorized dessert carts and specialty cookie/cupcake shops on every street corner. While people talk about exercising more than ever before, many people exercise on their way to fast food restaurants. Who could forget the image of former President Bill Clinton jogging to fast food restaurants? Others enjoy wearing exercise clothes, but participating is a different story. The same applies to living life without high-fat foods. For example, in a recent *Consumer Reports* article entitled "Are You Eating Right?" the editors noted that Americans were "still saying 'cheese'." That is, "Americans have soured on whole milk in the past thirty years and now choose low-fat milk more often. But consumption of high-fat cheeses has more than doubled in the same period, and even cream is rising."

Virtually all successful weight controllers consume much less fat than do average Americans. This means that they rarely eat most red meats, hardly ever eat desserts other than fruit or low-fat/no-fat alternatives (e.g., sorbet, frozen yogurt), and almost never eat fried foods. Their salad dressings are almost always fat-free and when they order salads in restaurants, they order salad dressings on the side. Some of my clients (and I) actually order barbeque sauce at restaurants and use that as a delicious salad dressing. They grill and broil and bake and steam foods, and they insist on being served foods prepared in those low-fat ways in restaurants. Successful weight controllers rarely eat anything with high-fat gravies or sauces. No-fat cheeses, ice cream, and mayonnaises are also among their possibilities. They think of normal-fat cookies, brownies, cake, and candy as foods for others (sometimes as "dog food"), not for themselves.

Many people really *do* live this way. For example, if you have made the change from whole milk to skim milk, do you miss drinking whole milk, or does it seem more like cream to you now? People find some of these changes easier to implement than you might expect. For example, consider the following comments from some of my more successful clients:

- "It's amazing, but I don't even want candy anymore. When I see candy, or people eating candy, I don't have the slightest interest in eating it."
- "I find fried foods disgustingly greasy now. Except for french fries, fried foods don't tempt me in the least. Okay, maybe onion rings tempt me a little, too."
- "This is the best time in history for living with fat-free and low-fat foods. There are so many perfectly good choices."
- "I now think of high fat-foods as 'alien foods.' I say to myself, 'that stuff is for people from other worlds.'"

Fat-Free Eating Tips. Some ideas about foods that have helped people make low-fat eating more palatable include substitutions for high-fat foods and suggestions for staples that appear in the Appendix of this book. Other ideas are:

- Snacks: air-popped popcorn, pretzels, fruit, rice cakes, sugar-free Jell-O, low-calorie cocoa, the usual raw vegetables (pre-peeled mini-carrots and sugar snap peas are especially good).
- Mustard on everything: collect, compare, and contrast many different varieties of mustards.
- Learn to love spicy foods.
- Salsa on everything: become a salsa connoisseur and collect, compare, and contrast many different varieties.
- Pasta, pasta, pasta.
- Tomato sauces: particularly low-fat versions.
- Fish, shellfish.
- Stir-fried cooking: use broths, water, no oil if possible.

- No-fat cheeses: try melting them on bagels or English muffins.
- Baked white or sweet-potatoes with non-fat sour cream, cottage cheese, or yogurt. Honey mustard works well, too, as a topping for potatoes.
- Soups: experiment with vegetables, beans, bones.
- Frozen entrees that specify amount of fat (e.g., Healthy Choice ravioli; Healthy Choice linguini with shrimp; Tyson roasted chicken; and Ultra Slim-Fast mesquite chicken).
- Canned no-fat soups.
- Use applesauce, and new oil and shortening replacement products made of fruit purees instead of butter and oil in baked goods—see Appendix for how to do these substitutions.
- Add fat-free broths, not oils, to marinades.
- Wrap fish in lettuce before baking to retain moisture. (Remove lettuce before serving—unless, of course, you love the taste of soggy, fishy lettuce!)
- To prevent yogurt from separating when heated, add one teaspoon of cornstarch for every cup of yogurt.
- Use yogurt or evaporated skim milk or cottage cheese instead of cream.
- Vegetable purees can thicken sauces. Mashed or pureed potatoes make a good thickener.
- Substitute two egg whites for one whole egg.
- Add vegetables or pastas to meat dishes to decrease the amount of meat (fat) per serving.

Certainly, nearly fat-free eating is very possible and very tasty. On the other hand, berries do not quite match the taste sensations of cheesecakes or chocolate mousses. Grilled swordfish may be a real treat, but it does not taste like a porterhouse steak. Unfortunately, high-fat food choices must become "alien food" to you, if you expect to lose weight and keep it off forever. You *can* do it. Many, many thousands of people have made the switch to very low-fat eating. It becomes a way of life and can be very satisfying. In any case, it beats the alternative for those of us who have lost weight. You cannot get to a lower weight and stay there without adopting a very low-fat eating plan.

The following "fat facts" underscore my emphasis on mastering this aspect of eating in order to lose weight and keep it off. Please review them carefully. If you know your enemy well (fat in this case), then you can defeat it more readily.

- Your body uses very little energy to digest and store high-fat foods (for example, three calories of energy expended to digest one hundred calories of bacon); your body uses much more energy to digest carbohydrates (twenty-two calories expended to digest one hundred calories of pasta).

- When you eat high-fat foods, the fat goes into storage very quickly—into your billions of hungry extra fat cells. When a never-overweight person eats high-fat foods, the fat goes into the muscles to be used as fuel.

- High-fat foods can cause an increase in appetite for more high-fat foods.

- Highly successful weight controllers report that their current successes, unlike prior weight losses, became permanent when they learned to eat very little fat.

- Goal for fat intake per day: as low as you can go. Aim for zero.

The following case provides an excellent example of how one of my clients focused her weight loss efforts on VLF eating. This focus led to great consistency and very satisfying long-term results.

Connie's Permanent Twenty Pound Weight Loss:
"It's My Body—That's the Way It Works."

Connie was sixty-one when I met her three years ago. She owns a successful, but very stressful, small business with twenty-seven employees, and is happily married to her second husband, who is in a similar line of work. She lived primarily in Chicago but spent a lot of time commuting to a distant suburb, where her ex-husband and their two grown daughters lived. She also did considerable traveling for work. In fact, she estimated that she ate approximately one-third her meals at restaurants.

Connie was quite happy in her work and with her second marriage (seven years at the time of our initial meeting). However, she was dissatisfied with her weight and fitness levels. She had been used to living her life as a trim, five-foot-four, 130-pound woman who was fairly athletic. Over the past ten years, however, as life had become more complex with more commuting and less available time, her exercising became more sporadic, and her weight increased by twenty-four pounds. Although she was not substantially overweight, and the health risks of this amount of excess weight were modest, it really bothered her a great deal to feel as though she was in a body, as she said, that "wasn't right for me."

Connie's main barriers to successful and permanent weight control were:

- Inconsistent exercise and sedentary living.
- Excessive drinking (one to two glasses of wine, sometimes much more, quite often).
- Often minimal eating early in the day or midday, with excessive eating in the evening.
- Some variability in consumption of fat (e.g., regular salad dressings on salads, bar food fairly often).

Connie had one perfect tendency for a weight controller: She liked looking at the details of her life. She was not at all adverse to self-monitoring, measuring, and focusing on exactly what she ate, how she moved, and the circumstances that affected her either positively or negatively. She did this religiously and enjoyed the process. She also began incorporating a more consistent eating pattern, beginning in the morning and including a modest lunch. She loved and sought out vegetable sandwiches, essentially salads between two slices of bread, usually with mustard as a condiment.

Connie did not focus directly on decreasing her drinking of an occasional beer or glass or wine, even though at times that might have been a problem. She didn't want to modify her drinking and believed she could incorporate it at a moderate level into a healthy lifestyle.

The following food records were obtained approximately six months after Connie started her program. She had already lost all twenty-two pounds by the time this example of her food record began. So, these records suggest what worked for Connie (and still works for her, five years after beginning this effort). You will note in these records that she ate very limited amounts of fat. That was a critical aspect of her success. What does not appear in these records, but was included in Connie's actual daily records, was her exercising. This included at least thirty minutes of exercise virtually every single day—generally walking, running, using a treadmill, some strength training, and various stretching and related exercises.

Take a look at these food records and consider what elements of Connie's approach you might incorporate into your own patterns. For example, you may wish to avoid using your calories for alcohol the way Connie does, but you might follow her example in minimizing your consumption of fat whenever and wherever possible.

MONDAY, JANUARY 6 / WEIGHT: 131.0		Calories	Fat Grams
7 a.m.	Coffee	25	0.5
	Banana/Orange Juice Shake	165	1.0
Noon	Fruit	200	1.0
7 p.m.	Rice	200	0.0
	Shrimp	90	1.0
	Salmon	120	5.0
	Pretzels	100	0.0
	Wine	270	0.0
	Milk	90	0.0
	Frozen Yogurt	120	0.0
Totals		1,380	8.5

TUESDAY, JANUARY 7 / WEIGHT: 130.0		Calories	Fat Grams
7:00 a.m.	Coffee	25	0.5
	Cereal	140	0.0
Noon	Veggie Sandwich	180	1.5
	Turkey, 1 slice	20	0.5
8 p.m.	Veggies	100	2.0
	Mashed sweet potatoes	200	1.0
	Rolls	60	0.5
	Pretzels	100	0.0
	Frozen Yogurt	120	0.0
	Milk	90	0.0
Totals		1,035	6.0

Saturday, October 11 / Weight: 130.0			
7:00 a.m.	Cereal	140	0.0
	Coffee	25	0.5
8:00 p.m.	Salad with clear rice noodles	100	0.0
	Wine	180	0.0
	Pretzels	100	0.0
	Frozen Yogurt	120	0.0
Totals		845	2.0

LOW CALORIC DENSITY: GETTING A BIGGER BANG FOR YOUR CALORIC BUCK

If you could eat as much as you wanted in order to feel satisfied, in which of the following meals would you wind up consuming more total calories?

Grilled chicken + seasoned white rice + assorted vegetables + one glass of ice water

Soup made from: grilled chicken, seasoned white rice, assorted vegetables, water

A variety of studies suggest that you would eat about twenty percent more food when presented in the usual fashion compared to the soup version. The soup version is low in energy density because the soup contains relatively few calories per ounce. You'd have consumed a good deal of the liquid from the soup when eating it. In contrast, the chicken dish with a glass of water on the side would produce higher caloric density in part because you wouldn't drink as much water during that meal. In everyday life, foods that are low in caloric density are foods that have low amounts of calories per gram or weight or per ounce in volume. These include vegetables, fruits, and very low-fat foods. Foods with the greatest caloric density would be such things as chocolate, pastries, and high-fat meats and cheeses.

Quite a few studies with animals and humans show that by adding more fluid to meals and decreasing the energy density accordingly, people eat considerably less than they do with the same fat levels at higher density presentations. Some of these studies also show that simply removing some high-density foods from a person's diet has little effect on their total consumption. On the other hand, removing all sources of high-fat foods almost always results in less eating overall, and eating much less fat.

Eating low-density foods increases the size of the stomach, and that creates a feeling of fullness. Eating such foods also slows down the rate of transfer of nutrients into the small intestines, another mechanism that decreases appetite and increases feelings of fullness.

A study of nearly 1,800 participants conducted in Philadelphia nicely illustrates this point. Greater consumption of soup was associated with better weight loss. Eating soup is a particularly good way of decreasing energy density levels in your diet. Perhaps similar findings would occur if the researchers measured consumption of salads per week or eating large portions of vegetables every day.

The take-away message from research on energy density is that you will find weight control easier if you focus on low-density foods. In particular, try to eat as much soup as you can, and order lots of vegetables when dining out. This will make you feel more satisfied more often, as well as decrease your desire to eat higher fat foods.

CALORIC CONTROL:
1,200-1,800 CALORIES PER DAY

If you ate unlimited quantities of very low-fat and even low-density foods, then you would certainly gain a substantial amount of weight. These two key elements of eating to lose weight can control your appetite and regulate your weight; however, you have to watch what happens on the scale as you implement this. If your activity levels have increased substantially, *and* you are following these food guidelines, but your weight doesn't change, then you have to consider focusing more specifically on the amount of calories you are consuming every day.

Highly successful weight controllers in a series of dozens of important studies of successful weight controllers (the National Weight Control Registry studies) have lost more than sixty pounds and maintained that weight loss for an average of six years. Their reported average intake per day is approximately 1,350 calories. Based on prior research that verifies reports of eating, it seems likely that this number is a bit low. Let's assume that their average intake is closer to 1,500 or 1,600 calories per day as a maintenance level. These numbers suggest that a good target for weight loss for most people might be 1,200 to 1,800 calories per day, in addition to considerable activity. Closer to 1,200 probably works best for most people, but some big, active people with higher metabolisms might do well on numbers as high as 1,800 calories per day. One study by psychologist Michael Perri and his colleagues at the University of Florida found that a 1,000 calorie per day goal produced better outcomes than a 1,500 calorie per day goal. One thousand calories per day seems too low to manage in the long run for most people, but using more stringent goals (e.g., 1,000, 1,200) can produce better results according to research on the effects of goal setting.

If you are able to lose weight consistently simply by following the other elements in this chapter and increasing your activity levels, then you can avoid targeting very low caloric consumption. That's pretty uncommon, however. Most people do better by including a specific caloric goal as part of their process toward success. One other caloric guideline also helps many people: *Consume no more than 800 calories at your biggest meal of the day.* This 800-calorie maximum per meal can help you when you're grappling with the menu at an Italian restaurant, for example. Many restaurants serve enormous portions of pasta that by themselves can greatly exceed 800 calories.

A recent report from the Centers for Disease Control shows why some attention to calorie consumption matters. According to this report, over the last thirty years, men have eaten 168 more calories daily than they did in 1971. They now eat, according to self-reports, approximately 2,600 calories a day. Women have consumed 335 more calories over these past thirty years, increasing their total calorie consumption to approximately 1,900 calories per day. Most nutritionists would argue that these self-reports are probably lower than reality. For example, a dietitian I know recently told me when discussing how much Americans actually consume these days, "We're now at the point that seven of ten Americans are either overweight or obese. We didn't get there on 1,900 to 2,600 calories per day. US food supply data indicate we're eating considerably more."

This means that if you are a serious weight controller, then you'll consume about half of what average Americans consume per day. You'll also expend far more energy than typical Americans, eat much less fat, and eat more low-density food. When you deviate so much from the average tendencies of those around you, you must rely on a good deal of inner strength to stay the course.

SECONDARY DIETARY PRINCIPLES

HOP's big three dietary principles make a huge difference when followed by weight controllers: eating very little fat, focusing on foods low in caloric density, and targeting 1,200 to 1,800 calories per day. In my previous books, I also emphasized four other dietary principles that can sometimes help quiet your appetite, and a final one that might help you maintain this approach forever.

The four secondary dietary principles that can decrease hunger are:

- **Protein**—Eating foods high in protein (e.g., egg whites, fat-free cheese, lean meats) especially early in the day, can decrease appetite. Protein acts as a time release capsule for hunger—lowering appetite over time better than any other nutrient. In the morning, your blood glucose level (stored energy) dips because you did not eat while sleeping. Quieting appetite via a good breakfast with a decent source of protein can work well.

- **Sugar**—Eating very sugary foods as stand-alone snacks (e.g., granola bars, fat-free cookies, sugary drinks) can increase your hunger level substantially. You can have frozen yogurt for dessert and not worry about it, but stand-alone sugary snacks do not work well for appetite control.

- **Drinking Your Calories**—Drinking your calories (e.g., juice, Gatorade, sugar-sweetened tea or soda) can increase your appetite and make achieving HOP's caloric goal for you quite difficult.

- **Fiber**—Foods high in fiber (non-digestible forms of fruits and vegetables, like whole grains, skin of fruit, and outer shells of beans) can help decrease hunger.

Here's the final point, a similar concept to the one I emphasized in several prior books, a tip about how to make your new eating lifestyle feel especially good and maximize your ability to sustain it forever: *Eat likeable foods that like you too.* In other words, to make this new eating pattern really work in the long run, seek out foods you really like but that also meet the standards for this program (e.g., very low in fat, low in caloric density). Weight controllers find such foods as baked sweet or white potatoes, veggie burgers, pizza with fat-free cheese, and frozen yogurt treats are examples of such lovable foods that love you back. This principle can increase your hunger, variety of food often does that, but the bigger picture seems to suggest that it makes this whole effort so much more pleasurable and sustainable. That makes the increase in appetite very worthwhile.

In my prior books, I worded this bit of encouragement to continue enjoying your food a bit differently: *Find lovable foods that love you back.* That invoked the concept of love as applied to food. One of the great mysteries of life concerns the ever-elusive meaning of the word love. The vast majority of songs written in the past century use this word, trying either to define it or encourage it. RET concepts argue against exaggeration in language. Using the word "like" instead may help calm down your enjoyment of food when trying to pursue this new lifestyle and healthy obsession. "Like" does that better than "love." After all, how can you deny yourself something you love? You can re-route your preferences for foods by focusing on liking what likes you (and your body) better than if you view foods as primary sources of love in your life. For example, consider how it feels when you say, "I really love ice cream!" Now try, "I really like chocolate frozen yogurt—and it likes me, too." The former creates an emotional bond with a very high-fat food. The latter promotes enjoyment of a similar food, but one that can work for you, not against you, in this new quest.

Two Key Questions. Ask yourself two key questions before eating anything to make this program work:

1. Is this food on my program?
2. Do I like it?

Hunger. Now, let's put appetite or hunger in proper perspective. Let's define hunger very simply: the desire for food. So, what impacts that desire for food? We just discussed several factors that impact hunger (e.g., drinking your calories, protein in the morning), but many others can work against you—or for you. Table 6-3 lists eighteen factors that research shows can affect hunger as we have defined it. Take a look at those factors and see if you agree.

HUNGRY?
The following factors influence the intensity of hunger (defined simply as "a desire for food"):
• Biology (e.g., fat cells)
• Eating by others (e.g., parties)
• Consumption of alcohol, marijuana, and other recreational drugs
• Emotions (e.g., stress, anger, frustration, boredom, etc.)
• Activities (e.g., exercise, amount of activity)
• Fat consumption
• Fiber
• Negative thoughts (e.g., "I've blown it already today.")
• Presence of foods, particularly highly appealing and attractive foods
• Protein consumption
• Stimuli that are associated with eating (e.g., in the car, while watching TV)
• Sugar consumption
• Talking about food
• Thinking about food
• Time of day and usual routines
• Tiredness
• Variety/blandness of diet
• Volume of food

TABLE 6-3

This list presents a cautionary tale. Eating control gets very complicated very fast. For example, when you exercise a lot, your immediate hunger usually goes down. But if you surround yourself with others who are eating high-fat foods (e.g., by taking a long walk to a bar to meet up with friends to watch a ballgame), you can reverse that typical effect of exercise and wind up stimulating your appetite. That's why Chapter 5 emphasized the vital role of a healthy obsession, and related, consistent self-monitoring. The three primary dietary principles can help you manage all of this, but nurturing a healthy obsession via careful self-monitoring can help you stay focused despite the complex ways that the world can fight against your efforts. Appendix 1 provides other useful tidbits on how to shop and cook using a very low-fat approach.

EATING AND CANCER: CAN YOU PREVENT CANCER BY EATING BETTER?

Cancer strikes ten million people a year. Three to four million of those cancers could have been prevented through healthier eating and exercising. In fact, eating more fruits and vegetables alone could eliminate as many as two million new cases of cancer a year.

Recently, The World Cancer Research Fund and the American Institute for Cancer Research formed a panel that issued a comprehensive report on the relationship between eating and cancer. This report, based on a careful review of more than 4,500 studies, stressed that no food or drink can prevent cancer, but concluded that a diet that emphasizes certain foods can certainly lower your risk of getting this deadly disease.

In addition to decreasing consumption of animal protein, based on the research described by Dr. T. Colin Campbell in *The China Study*, five eating and drinking strategies that can decrease the risk of getting cancer are:

1. **Eat lots of vegetables.** The average American eats only three or four servings a day of vegetables and fruits. Five servings are clearly preferable, and nine are recommended by virtually all nutritional experts. Yellow, dark green, and orange vegetables rich in carotenoids, and all the cabbage family vegetables (broccoli, Brussels sprouts, cauliflower, collards, kale, bok choy, and mustard/turnip greens) all seem to lower the risk of cancer. Garlic, onions, and leeks may also help ward off cancer, especially breast cancer.

2. **Eat Lots of fruits.** Fruits that are rich in vitamin C (all citrus fruits, tomatoes, and strawberries) are especially helpful.

3. **Decrease consumption of total FAT, particularly saturated fat.** This panel recommended that fats should provide between fifteen and thirty percent of total calories. You may recall that I have recommended that you go "as low as you can go" in total fat. For most, this will amount to less than ten percent of your total calories in fat.

4. **Decrease alcohol consumption; limit drinks to less than two a day for men and one a day for women.** The panel concluded that although alcohol may have some benefits for decreasing heart disease when consumed in small amounts, the risk for cancers, particularly breast, colon, and rectal cancers, is significant. People who consume even small amounts of alcohol show a significantly greater chance of developing cancer than those who do not drink alcohol at all.

5. The following other foods and drinks may also help reduce the risk of cancer, at least somewhat:
    - dried beans
    - milk
    - fish
    - green tea
    - whole-grain
    - cereals
    - olive oil

The evidence favoring these particular foods and drinks is not as convincing as the evidence in the first four recommendations. Nonetheless, the panel concluded that those items may prove beneficial and are worth including in healthy eating plans. Olive oil, however, does not fit in this program (i.e., fourteen fat grams per tablespoon makes it a very high-fat food).

SUMMARY AND CONCLUSIONS

Table 6-4 summarizes the three key principles of eating. Focusing on consuming as little fat as possible will help you implement the other two elements. When you eat a very low-fat diet, you will naturally gravitate to low caloric-density foods because fat is by far the most calorically dense nutrient (nine calories per gram versus four calories per gram for protein and carbs). Decreasing fat also leads to eating relatively few total calories. Low-density and very low-fat foods also have lots of fiber, and so on. So, start your focus with the goal of near zero fat intake and you'll get to the most healthful diet over time, including foods you like that like you too. This approach clearly does not focus on moderation. Moderation simply does not work for weight controllers.

Fat Intake:

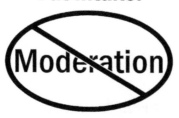

THREE KEYS TO EATING TO LOSE WEIGHT
1. VLF: Eat Very Low Fat: aim for zero grams.
2. Consume Low Caloric-Density Foods: e.g., lots of soups, fruits, and vegetables.
3. Caloric Control: Target 1,200-1,800 calories per day.

TABLE 6-4

CHAPTER 7

HOP Step 4: Maximizing Movement

Do any of the following benefits of movement surprise you?

Activity can:

- Increase weight loss
- Improve maintenance of weight loss
- Improve stress management
- Improve quality of sleep
- Improve digestion
- Improve metabolism of fat
- Enhance self-esteem
- Improve resistance to illness
- Increase energy levels
- Reduce blood pressure
- Increase flexibility
- Increase metabolic rate
- Build strength
- Decrease depression
- Increase endorphins (internally produced opiates that improve feelings of well-being and mood)
- Decrease appetite
- Increase life span

Most people find this list impressive but still fail to act on it. In fact, the single greatest predictor of long-term success in weight control is activity level. But most adults in North America do not get nearly enough activity to produce many of these health, emotional, or hedonic benefits. In fact, only twenty percent of adults over the age of twenty-five engage in physical activity at least twice per week.

Perhaps the most remarkable thing about the benefits of activity is that weight controllers don't have to exercise in the traditional sense in order to get most of these benefits. The most common activity is just plain walking, and studies of successful weight controllers reveal that they prefer this form of activity: the average master of weight control walks briskly for one hour each day.

The best thing about walking is it doesn't require a gym membership or a nearby club or sports team, just putting one foot in front of the other. Let's consider in more detail how you can get yourself to move more consistently in this simple way, by taking more steps every day.

KEY GOAL: 12,000+ STEPS A DAY

At Wellspring Camps, most of the teenage participants scoffed at 12,000 steps. Wellspring campers averaged a remarkable 24,000 steps per day. About 2,000 steps equals a mile and adults average 4,000 steps per day. But most of that comes from just everyday activities, not from deliberate efforts to get to the goal. The difference between a goal of 12,000 and a daily average of 4,000 from everyday activities is about 8,000 steps per day. That's about an hour or so of *additional* walking each day, less time if the activity involves moving faster than walking.

Buying Pedometers, Downloading Step Apps, or Using Fitbits

Pedometers are remarkable devices that sit on your hip and count each step you take. Some cheaper pedometers (less than $10) do this with a spring mechanism that may not measure steps accurately. The better pedometers involve a sensitive ball-like mechanism that moves up and down with your stride, as the elevation of your hip changes ever so slightly. More high-tech versions appear now as apps on all smart phones (e.g., Strava) and via remarkable devices that you can wear as a bracelet and download information about steps taken, calories burned, time spent in sedentary behaviors, and even time of day (e.g., Nike+ Apple Watch, www.Nike.com).

Wearing a pedometer (or related device) can provide you with critical and immediate feedback about your progress relative to the daily goal of 12,000 steps. The pedometer revolution started in Japan about forty years ago and made its way to the US and Canada after researchers at the Cooper Clinic in Dallas demonstrated their importance in promoting activity. You can get an accurate pedometer for about $20, such as those made by Kenz, Accusplit, Yamax, and New Lifestyles (see www.accusplit.com and www. omronhealthcare.com). Most pedometer-like apps are free, and Fitbits and related products cost $60 to $300.

How about getting all members of your family to use step apps? If everyone does this, tracking steps will become the new normal—an important goal for the whole family. Family members will endorse parking further away from destinations or using stairs instead of the elevator just to get more steps. The research on the use of pedometers demonstrates these effects; just wearing them increases steps by about forty percent, and wearing them after setting goals increases steps even more (eighty percent).

The Advantages of Focusing on Steps

The focus on steps uses the KISSeS principle—Keep It Scientific, Simple, and Sustainable. The goal of 12,000 steps also meets all three S's.

- **SCIENTIFIC:** Successful weight controllers move a lot more than average people. In general, maintaining a high level of activity helps maintain weight loss more than any other single factor that has been studied. For example, psychologist Ross Andersen and his colleagues from Johns Hopkins University School of Medicine followed thirty-three overweight women through sixteen weeks of a structured cognitive-behavioral treatment program and then for one year after the program ended. The women lost an average of eighteen pounds during treatment, but more importantly, the group that reported relatively high activity levels after treatment fared far better than the least active group during the one-year follow-up. This more active one-third of the participants, on average, achieved the goal of at least thirty minutes of activity per day at least five of seven days per week for seventy-nine percent of the weeks during the follow-up year. This group continued losing weight during the follow-up period. This level of activity is quite possibly 10,000-plus steps per day, close to the 12,000 steps per day goal in HOP. The least active third of participants in the study achieved that goal during only nineteen percent of the weeks in the follow-up period and, as you might expect, on average they regained most of the weight that they had lost during treatment. Figure 7-1 summarizes these important results.

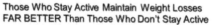

Those Who Stay Active Maintain Weight Losses
FAR BETTER Than Those Who Don't Stay Active

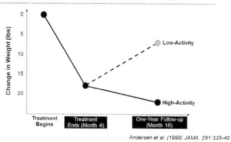

Andersen et al. (1999) JAMA. 281:335-40.

- <u>**SIMPLE:**</u> Simple behavioral directives provide clear direction for actions, easily measured goals, and readily available feedback about progress. Wearing a step counting device provides great feedback, especially because feeling it on your wrist or looking at it over the course of the day helps remind weight controllers about their commitment. The direction for action and the goal are certainly clear and measurable: Walk enough to reach 12,000 on your pedometer every day.

- **SUSTAINABLE:** Walking is the preferred form of activity for most people. Walkers and runners actually move more and at higher intensities (faster) when listening to music. Many families walk together, shop together, and use this very natural form of movement to create more active lifestyles.

Sitting versus Standing versus Moving

The following table also helps make the point about the critical role of steps. Take a look at the differences between "sitting or lying down" versus "standing quietly" versus "walking fast." Standing up expends twenty percent more energy than sitting down. Walking fast expends more than 300 percent more energy than sitting down.

SITTING VS. STANDING VS. MOVING: CALORIES EXPENDED PER MINUTE	
Sitting or lying down	2.0 calories per minute
Standing quietly	2.4 calories per minute
Walking fast (4 mph)	8.2 calories per minute
Running (9 min. mile)	17.6 calories per minute

Even shopping expends almost three times more energy as sitting, as long as you keep moving. (Then when you buy something, at least you get the benefit of standing, a twenty percent boost in energy expenditure over sitting.)

Some adult weight controllers even purchase desks that allow them to stand up just to get that extra twenty percent energy expenditure. It also helps to know how to equate activities and sports to steps. The following tables should be helpful.

STEP EQUIVALENTS PER MINUTE (HIERARCHIAL)	
Activity	Equivalent # of Steps Per Minute of Activity
Bowling	55
Cycling (5 mph)	55
Dancing (slow)	55
Shopping	60
Walking (2 mph)	60
Canoeing (2.5 mph)	70
Golfing (with cart)	70
Volleyball (leisurely)	70
Rowing (leisurely)	75
Vacuuming	75
Washing the car	75
Window cleaning	75
Painting	80
Walking (3 mph)	80
Mopping	85
Gardening (moderate)	90
Housework	90
Table tennis	90
Ice skating (leisurely)	95
Dancing (non-contact)	100
Golfing (no cart)	100
Walking (4 mph)	100
Waxing the car	100

Tennis (doubles)	110
Aerobic dancing (low impact)	115
Swimming (25 yards/min.)	120
Volleyball game	120
Bicycling (10 mph)	125
Weight training (90 seconds b/w sets)	125
Basketball (leisurely, non-game)	130
Skiing (downhill)	130
Mowing lawn	135
Scrubbing floor	140
Stair climbing	140
Aerobics, step training (4" step)	145
Badminton	150
Roller skating (moderate)	150
Cross-country Skiing (leisurely)	155
Gardening (heavy)	155
Hiking (no load)	155
Stairmaster	160
Tennis (singles)	160
Water skiing	160
Ice skating (competitive)	170
Dancing (fast)	175
Hiking (10 lb. load)	180
Rowing machine	180
Running (5 mph)	185
Judo (competitive)	185
Aerobics (intense)	190

Scuba diving	190
Weight training (60 seconds b/w sets)	190
Snow shoveling	195
Soccer (competitive)	195
Cycling (12 mph)	200
Elliptical machine (moderate)	200
Racquetball	205
Squash	205
Cross-country skiing (moderate)	220
Basketball (game)	220
Swimming (50 yards/min.)	225
Handball	230
Jogging (6 mph)	230
Hiking (30 lb. load)	235
Weight training (40 seconds b/w sets)	255
Elliptical (fast)	270
Skipping rope	285
Swimming (75 yards/min.)	290
Running (8 mph)	305
Cross-country skiing (fast)	330
Running (10 mph)	350

Step Equivalents Per Minute (Alphabetical Listing)

Activity	Equivalent # of Steps Per Minute of Activity
Aerobic dancing (low impact)	115
Aerobics (intense)	190
Aerobics step training (4″ step)	145
Badminton	150
Basketball (game)	220
Basketball (leisurely, non-game)	130
Bicycling (10 mph)	125
Bowling	55
Canoeing (2.5 mph)	70
Cross-country skiing (fast)	330
Cross-country skiing (leisurely)	155
Cross-country skiing (moderate)	220
Cycling (12 mph)	200
Cycling (5 mph)	55
Dancing (fast)	175
Dancing (non-contact)	100
Dancing (slow)	55
Elliptical machine (fast)	270
Elliptical machine (moderate)	200
Gardening (heavy)	155
Gardening (moderate)	90
Golfing (no cart)	100
Golfing (with cart)	70
Handball	230

Hiking (10 lb. load)	180
Hiking (30 lb. load)	235
Hiking (no load)	155
Housework	90
Ice skating (competitive)	170
Ice skating (leisurely)	95
Jogging (6 mph)	230
Judo (competitive)	185
Mopping	85
Mowing lawn	135
Painting	80
Racquetball	205
Roller skating (moderate)	150
Rowing (leisurely)	75
Rowing machine	180
Running (10 mph)	350
Running (5 mph)	185
Running (8 mph)	305
Scrubbing floor	140
Scuba diving	190
Shopping	60
Skiing (downhill)	130
Skipping rope	285
Snow shoveling	195
Soccer (competitive)	195
Squash	205
Stair climbing	140
Stairmaster	160
Swimming (25 yards/min.)	120
Swimming (50 yards/min.)	225

Swimming (75 yards/min.)	290
Table tennis	90
Tennis (doubles)	110
Tennis (singles)	160
Vacuuming	75
Volleyball (leisurely)	70
Volleyball game	120
Walking (2 mph)	60
Walking (3 mph)	80
Walking (4 mph)	100
Washing the car	75
Water skiing	160
Waxing the car	100
Weight training (40 seconds b/w sets)	255
Weight training (60 seconds b/w sets)	190
Weight training (90 seconds b/w sets)	125
Window cleaning	75

Strategies for Reaching 12,000 Steps

Get Up Early. Early mornings are the only time of day we all can control. Over many decades, I discovered that of my very successful weight controllers, about ninety percent got most of their steps in the early morning hours. Those who work out later often get distracted by their lives and skip far too many days accordingly

Walk to Watch. One of the more noteworthy innovations at Wellspring's former boarding schools was the requirement that students had to be on a treadmill, elliptical, stationery bike, or Stairmaster in order to watch TV. This will be too much for most families to enforce.

However, what about purchasing at least one piece of fitness equipment for the room where most television is watched? If you're buying one, consistent with our focus on walking, you'll do better with a treadmill—not an elliptical or a bike or some even fancier machine that claims it burns even more calories per minute of use. The key word in the last sentence is use: treadmills get used much more than other fitness equipment.

Putting a treadmill in front (hopefully directly in front) of the television is an important step for promoting steps. It helps to have many channels and the capability of watching movies in front of such machines.

Getting Steps in Many Ways: Dimensions of Movement

Although getting 12,000 steps per day is the key to long-term weight control, it's also important to consider some other aspects of being active. At Wellspring, families asked some great questions about movement. Consider your answer to the following:

- Does it matter if my daughter does the same form of exercise every day?
- Isn't variety both the spice of life and the thing that helps kids stay motivated to be active?
- Walking doesn't seem like real exercise to me. Don't you have to break a sweat to help you lose weight?
- I've heard many trainers talk about the value of taking a rest day at least once a week. Is that a good idea? It seems inconsistent with the concept of Healthy Obsession.

The American College of Sports Medicine (ACSM) has provided recommendations to answer these questions. ACSM consists of many of the world's leading experts on activity. ACSM's most recent set of recommendations has become accepted around the world as the basis for developing safe and effective activity patterns.

Let's review answers to commonly asked questions by considering five aspects of activity and the ACSM recommendations that pertain to each one. These aspects are:

- Frequency of activity
- Intensity of activity
- Duration of activity
- Variety of activity
- Strength training

Frequency of Activity. The goal is 12,000 steps every single day. Not every other day or even six days a week. Consistency can make a huge difference for weight controllers. Masters of weight control who participated in the National Weight Control Registry studies report about one hour's worth of brisk walking each day. These people know that activity every day helped them succeed.

In terms of biology, daily activity helps prevent the negative effects of what is sometimes called "the desert island effect" on metabolism. When weight controllers reduce food intake and lose weight, the body reacts by lowering the metabolic rate. The metabolic rate is the amount of energy our bodies expend to keep us alive at rest. This includes energy to keep the heart pumping and the liver working to break down the food we eat and transfer the energy from the food into our cells. Even active people expend more energy on these bodily functions operating twenty-four hours (86,400 seconds) per day than they expend for movement and exercise. So, metabolic rate matters a great deal. When the body detects a reduction in food intake, it "thinks" something like, *"Uh oh, I've got to conserve energy to keep this person alive."* Remember, humans survived as hunter-gatherers for tens of thousands of years, and evolution caused our bodies to adapt by lowering our metabolic rate when we had trouble finding enough food. This metabolic shift helped us survive much longer during famines. This effect is called the "desert island effect." If you found yourself abandoned on a desert island, this metabolic shift might save your life by allowing you to survive with relatively few calories.

Staying active every day allows weight controllers to reverse the desert island effect. The first study on this, in 1984, showed that about thirty minutes of brisk walking can keep the metabolic rate in a normal range despite lowered caloric intake of food. This finding has been confirmed in many studies over the past thirty-plus years. Interestingly, our ability to reverse the desert island effect with activity only lasts about twenty-four hours. In other words, to keep the metabolic rate normal and make weight loss easier, weight controllers must stay active virtually every day, not just a few, or even most, days of the week.

Another important reason for the daily goal is that it is simpler, clearer, and more difficult to rationalize non-compliance, and much more effective. With a daily goal, it's hard to make excuses to avoid activity. This contrasts with a five-day-a-week goal, where most people will wind up saying to themselves: "Today is the day I won't exercise. I'll exercise tomorrow." This kind of thinking tends to result in skipping one day after another, and then abandonment.

Intensity of Activity. Intensity refers to how hard your body works over a period of time. More intensive activity means the body works harder for the fifteen or thirty or forty-five minutes when you're active. Intensity varies depending on one's level of conditioning or fitness. For example, world-class marathoners can run three eight-minute miles in a row without breaking a sweat. To the average person, this intensity would prove extremely challenging. The most important rule of thumb about intensity is this: Keep the intensity low enough to allow yourself to be active comfortably for at least thirty minutes per session.

Duration of Activity. The ACSM endorses activity sessions lasting from thirty to sixty minutes. However, some overweight people have difficulty maintaining aerobic activity for thirty minutes or more. If this describes you, try starting with sessions that last ten or fifteen minutes. Two fifteen-minute sessions of exercise produce about the same benefits as one thirty-minute session.

Some confusing notions exist about required duration of activity. One concerns "fat burning," suggesting you won't "burn fat" unless you're active for an extended period. This assertion is wrong. When you begin activity, you begin using calories immediately. Initially, the energy consumed by your body comes from glucose stored in the muscles. As you exercise for longer periods of time, your body begins dipping into its energy reserves (fat). However, your body must replenish the energy supply it uses. This means that when you consume energy in the form of stored glucose from the muscles, your body will use its stored energy supply to replenish the glucose taken from the muscles. It makes no difference whether you're active for short bursts of ten or fifteen minutes or for longer periods of thirty to sixty minutes per session. Both ways burn fat.

Duration can help you much more than intensity for weight control. Consider how to get the most steps. If you walk for an hour, you'll get between 6,000 and 8,000 steps. If you run as hard as you can for as long as you can and only go for four minutes, you'll get about 1,000 steps. Keep this comparison in mind to remember that anything you do that involves movement of any kind works far better than doing very intense activities that can prove frustrating and exhausting.

Variety of Activity. Imagine what would happen if you fed your dog Fido some brand new Super Chow. Assuming this dog chow tastes great—and because it's very low-fat, you can bet that it does—when you serve him the first bowl, he gobbles it down right away. Then he glances at you with those begging eyes hoping for another bowl. After a month or two, you notice that the Super Chow sits in Fido's bowl for half the day, barely touched. He eats it eventually, but the gusto is gone. Then you switch him back to what he used to eat—Brand X. You're a bit surprised to see that Fido is chomping down on Brand X with the same gusto he used to have for Super Chow. After a month or so on Brand X, Fido's interest in this chow declines. The first day you re-introduce Super Chow, the gusto returns.

You've heard the expression "variety is the spice of life." So it is with Fido. And so it is with weight controllers, particularly novice weight controllers. In terms of getting 12,000 steps, variety adds excitement and increases the probability of achieving this important goal.

Strength Training (Weight Lifting). Beginning in 1990, ACSM recognized and emphasized the importance of resistance training more than in any of their previous recommendations. Strength training of moderate intensity (fifty to sixty percent of maximum lifting ability) provides important benefits. In particular, strength training can prevent injuries and reshape the body in favorable ways.

ACSM recommends selecting exercises that incorporate many different body parts and different kinds of movements. They suggest performing lifting exercises continuously, using smooth, slow, and controlled motions. Maintaining a good posture while lifting also helps avoid injury. Only the body part being exercised while lifting the weight should be in motion during a lift. Other body parts should be at rest and stationary when weight lifting.

The following box shows some frequently asked questions and answers about strength training.

FREQUENTLY ASKED QUESTIONS ABOUT STRENGTH TRAINING

How many repetitions? Eight to twelve repetitions improve both strength and endurance. Most exercise experts suggest that if you can lift the weight easily more than twelve times, it is time to add more weight. When you add more weight, go back to eight to twelve repetitions per exercise.

How many sets? The ACSM recommends using eight to ten different kinds of weight-lifting exercises per set. If you only make time to do one set, you will still strengthen your muscles seventy to eighty percent as much as you would by doing multiple sets. Two sets yields about ninety-five percent of the maximum benefit and three sets creates the full benefit or one hundred percent. A full set of eight or ten lifting exercises, including warm-up time, can take as little as fifteen minutes to do.

How many workouts? The ideal strengthening program includes three workouts a week. Squeezing in more than three workouts per week might slow the growth of your muscles. Muscles may need some time off to recover from weight training. Interestingly, you can get about seventy-five percent of the maximum improvement available from weight lifting by working out only twice a week. If you don't have much time, even a single strengthening session per week helps far more than none at all. According to one study, a weekly workout can maintain current levels of strength for several months.

How much is enough? To keep building strength, you must keep increasing the weights you lift. You can maintain a desired level of strength by simply maintaining twelve repetitions for a particular exercise. If you stop weight lifting, your strength will begin to fade within two weeks. After three to five months, you'll be back to where you started. *What's the procedure for weight lifting?* Several guidelines can help prevent injuries and maximize the benefits of weight lifting.

1. It helps to warm up for a few minutes by walking briskly or jogging in place, and then do stretching exercises. It helps to stretch your shoulders, lower back, calves, and front and back of the thighs. Stretch slowly and steadily to the point of tension, not pain, and hold the position for three to thirty seconds.

2. Breathe slowly and steadily during weight lifting. Holding your breath while tensing muscles can cause light-headedness and even fainting. Exhale as you either lift the weight or raise your body, and inhale as you return to the starting position.

3. Perform the repetitions slowly. Each one should take about six seconds—two to lift and four to lower. Jerky movements can cause injury and soreness.

4. Stop if your muscles hurt. The dictum "No pain, no gain" is both wrong and potentially dangerous. Your muscles should feel fatigued during the last repetitions, but you should not feel sharp or piercing pains in your muscles. If you do feel pain, stop the exercise immediately.

5. Cool down after you exercise by doing a few minutes of walking or light jogging, followed by stretching again.

Taking the Next Step: Planning

The following example was developed by one of my clients for a recent Thanksgiving break. Notice the level of detail and major facets of the plan, including a component focused on problem solving. The key is to focus on how to achieve 12,000-plus steps—regardless of the time of year or obstacles in the way. This can go a long way toward permanent success.

Goals & Plans for the Thanksgiving Break

1. STEPS PER DAY—GOALS:
Minimum Level: 12,000
Average: 15,000
PLANS:
- ✔ Morning Pandora App walk, 45 min.
- ✔ Walk the dog in the eve, 20 min.
- ✔ Keep moving whenever possible
- ✔ No escalators or elevators when shopping

2. WORKOUT ACTIVITIES—GOALS:
Resistance bands every day; 2/4 days workout
PLANS:
- ✔ YMCA with a friend at least once
- ✔ YMCA total at least twice
- ✔ Bands in the am every day

3. MINIMIZING SEDENTARY BEHAVIORS—GOALS:
Three hours per day max on TV and computer
PLANS:
- ✔ I'll shop, bowl, whatever every day—be sure to hit my step goals.

4. SOURCES OF ENCOURAGEMENT:
- ✔ I'll text a friend at least once a day about how it's going.
- ✔ I'll bring the CalorieKing book and read at least something in it every day.
- ✔ I'll talk plenty with my family about this.

5. METHODS OF PROBLEM SOLVING
- ✔ I'll self-monitor and journal every day.
- ✔ I'll be honest with myself if I get in trouble or really upset, then get consultation from a friend about it.

CHAPTER 8

HOP STEP 5: CREATING A SUPPORTIVE WORLD AROUND YOU

People with strong relationships suffer fewer medical and emotional problems than those who are more isolated. A study of 7,000 adults in California showed that people who lacked strong relationships with others died at a younger age than those who had strong relationships (i.e., married, frequent contacts with friends and neighbors, belonged to social clubs or religious groups).

Many other studies demonstrate that support from others can reduce the effects of stressors:

- Women who had a companion with them during labor and childbirth experience fewer complications than women who gave birth alone. Women in the supported group gave birth sooner, were awake more after delivery, and played more with their babies.

- Social support helps men who lose their jobs. Men with good support report fewer illnesses and less depression than men who do not have adequate support.

- Recovery from heart attacks is improved with the support of spouses, friends, and relatives.

Simply put, we do better at almost anything when we're surrounded by people who actively show they care. Most athletes certainly know this. Elite athletes build their own teams in many sports, sometimes including personal coaches, trainers, sport psychologists, and managers. Let's consider the types of support available to you, the types of coaches that athletes seek, and what you can do to create your best winning team.

Types of Support

You can benefit from three types of support: emotional, informational, and material support. You've undoubtedly used all of them at some points in your life.

EMOTIONAL SUPPORT. Others provide emotional support to you when they:
- Listen and talk things over with you, showing you understanding or empathy.
- Show confidence in you and provide encouragement.

INFORMATIONAL SUPPORT. People provide you with informational support when they:
- Give you worthwhile advice.
- Provide you with resources that prove useful.
- Suggest various solutions to problems from which you can choose courses of action.

MATERIAL SUPPORT. Material support from others sometimes comes in various forms, like:

- Food
- Money
- Shelter
- Clothing
- Education

Because the support of friends and family can play such an important role in managing the challenges of life, one great stress management skill is knowing when and who to ask for help. Complete Exercise 8-1 to consider those that you can rely on to help you manage the challenges you face in your life.

Exercise 8-1 Sources of Support in My Life

Instructions: *Just fill in the blanks and see who emerges as your supportive friends, colleagues, and family members.*

People that...	At Home	At Work	At Play
Calm me			
Bring me joy			
Make me laugh			
Listen to me			
Really care about me			
Provide me with material support when requested			
Challenge me, but in a good way			
Help me think through possible solutions to problems			
Energize me			
Seem to know amazing amounts of information			

Some of these supportive people in your life might want advice about how to support you most effectively in your quest to lose weight permanently. You can show them the suggestions in Table 8-1 to guide them.

How to Support a Weight Controller's Efforts

Losing weight and keeping it off is a very difficult process. You can make it easier for your spouse, friend, or partner. Here are several suggestions that will help you support and encourage the weight controllers in your life.

General Attitude

Be positive. Convey to the weight controller that even though it is very difficult to control weight, you believe he or she can do it. This attitude will boost the person's self-confidence while acknowledging the difficulties. Avoid negative comments, criticism, and coercion. These are unhelpful and demoralizing, and will create negative feelings between you and the weight controller. This, in turn, could cause him or her to eat more—not less—and thwart the likelihood of success in the long run.

Be reinforcing. Acknowledge the weight controller's accomplishments. Compliments, attention, encouragement, and tangible reinforcement (like little gifts) can help him or her stay motivated and adhere to the plan. Remember, be sincere; superficiality will be interpreted as condescending.

Be realistic. Weight control requires tremendous effort and skill to overcome strong biological forces. People who are trying to lose weight must adopt eating and exercise patterns that are much more stringent than normal. Don't expect the weight controller to be perfect, or even close to perfect. Occasional slips of overeating, inactivity, weight gain, and failure to adhere to plans will occur. Help the weight controller learn from these experiences rather than dwell on them as "failures."

Communicate. Occasionally inquire about the weight controller's progress. Ask him or her how you can help, thereby complimenting the weight controller's individual efforts. Be open to discussing the challenges of weight control and to assist in solving problems.

Managing Food

Increase the amount of nutritious, low-fat foods available to the weight controller.

Do NOT encourage the weight controller to eat foods that he or she is trying to avoid. For example, refrain from saying, "Let's go out for ice cream," or "Oh, come on, a little bit isn't going to hurt you."

Help the weight controller prepare foods and recipes in a low-fat way. Encourage experimentation and adventure.
Adopt appropriate eating habits, for example: not eating when full; eating appropriate portions; eating in a slow, deliberate fashion; eating regularly or on a schedule; limiting snacking; and limiting the number of eating situations. You may not have a weight problem, but better eating habits may improve your health, too, and will support the weight controller's efforts.
Plan activities with the weight controller that do not revolve around food (for example, sporting events, concerts, games).
When you go to a restaurant with the weight controller, select places that make low-fat/low-sugar eating as pleasant as possible.
Promoting Exercise
Plan activities with the weight controller that involve exercise (for example, walking, hiking, sports).
Become an exercise partner. You will reap the same physical benefits as your partner.
Support and encourage the weight controller's individual efforts to exercise.

Types of Coaches: Lessons Learned by Athletes

One of the best coaches of all time, legendary UCLA basketball coach John Wooden, the "Wizard of Westwood," won an unprecedented ten of twelve NCAA basketball championships. He emphasized effort more than winning and support/encouragement more than control:

"You cannot find a player who ever played for me that can tell you that he ever heard me mention winning a basketball game ... The last thing that I told my players, just prior to tipoff, [was] 'When the game is over, I want your head up—and I know of only one way for your head to be up—and that's for you to know that you did your best ... this means to do the best YOU can do. That's the best; no one can do more ... you made that effort'."

—SMITH, 1993, P.31

Very few coaches produce the kind of loyalty and intense admiration that virtually all of his players had for John Wooden. Very few athletes have a chance to play with such a legendary coach. But athletes often have choices about their coaches. What do they look for in a coach? How do the best coaches help their athletes? Research on coaching styles, athlete preferences, and effective coaching techniques provide answers to these important questions.

Coaching Styles. Research has identified three types of coaching styles. As you review them, consider which one you might prefer in someone who could help you as a trainer or weight-control counselor/therapist.

- *Task-oriented vs. Relationship-oriented.* Task-oriented coaches work together with athletes to get the job done. They focus on training and instruction. They attempt to improve the performance of their athletes by providing good technical instruction on skills, techniques, and strategies. They emphasize and facilitate rigorous training. When players make errors, they focus on corrective, technical advice.

  Relationship-oriented coaches focus more on developing interpersonal relationships between themselves and their athletes and within teams. They keep lines of communication open and maintain positivity in their connections to their athletes. They focus on how athletes feel, focusing more on feelings and team spirit than on technical aspects of their sports.

- *Democratic vs. Autocratic.* A democratic decision-making style allows athletes to participate in decisions. These coaches sometimes have athletes help decide the team's goals, practice techniques and schedules, and game plans—to varying extents. In contrast, the autocratically oriented coach remains aloof from athletes. These coaches stress their authority in making the team work and tend to seem powerful and intimidating.

- *Supportive vs. Punitive.* Coaches who focus on support show concern for the welfare of each of their athletes. They attempt to establish warm, personal relationships with fewer boundaries off the playing field than most other types of coaches. They also emphasize the good in their athletes via positive reinforcement whenever possible. In contrast, some coaches use a punitive style which involves more critical comments and harshness toward the players. These coaches maintain rigid boundaries off the field. Perhaps the idea behind this emphasis is "spare the rod and spoil the child."

Athletes generally prefer more supportive and democratic coaching styles. However, circumstances can significantly affect these preferences. For example, as athletes get older and develop higher levels of skill, they tend to prefer more task-oriented and autocratic coaching styles. Also, athletes who themselves are more social and relationship-oriented tend to perform better with coaches who emphasize such things. Another very logical differentiator pertains to the nature of the sport. Athletes who play very interactive large-scale complex team sports like football and volleyball tend to prefer more autocratic styles than athletes who play individual sports like golf or bowling or tennis. This makes sense. More autocratic styles create more efficient and focused leadership. A democratic style in a highly complex team sport can cause confusion.

Lessons Learned. In addition to the pattern of preferences for coaches of different styles, athletes look for effectiveness of the coach. They want coaches who win. Winning coaches succeed because of skills in recruitment, reputation, and knowledge of the sport, and how best to teach and execute.

For weight controllers, some parallels in understanding could help you achieve your goals. For example, you can rely on measures of effectiveness just as athletes do. In your case, you'd want to get involved with programs and people who have demonstrated their effectiveness. Those demonstrations appear in scientific journals and reputations among respected professional referral sources. If deciding to attend programs or seek professional help, the following section will provide some useful guidance. You would also want to select leaders of the programs or consultation to match your knowledge and skill level as a weight controller. For example, if you've tried Weight Watchers several times before, you're not likely to find that useful at this stage in your program. More individualized consultation from higher level experts or programs would suit you better, just as more experienced athletes prefer different coaching styles than their inexperienced peers.

Creating Your Team: Structure Works

Athletes frequently develop structure around them, essentially their own support teams. Team members include coaches, training buddies, personal trainers (strength, conditioning, sport specific), and sometimes sport psychologists. They rely on these support teams to keep them focused, exactly what weight controllers struggle to maintain quite often. Studies of sport psychology and weight management show that tremendous benefits accrue by adding effective support teams around both athletes and weight controllers. Adding structure can range from simple changes to substantial and potentially more powerful interventions. Let's consider the major options for your support team.

Get a Little Help from Your Friends. Supportive friends can help you by working out with you, staying on the plan you adopt from this book themselves, supporting you when you eat on plan, helping you problem solve if you hit a rough patch, and in many other ways. These friends also stand to benefit by helping you. Many people want to increase their thinness and fitness. You can show them how to reach those goals, as they help you reach yours.

Other Structured Assists. Personal trainers can help you stay focused and motivated. Most health clubs will only hire people with certifications from various recognized organizations, like the American Council of Sports Medicine (ASCM) and the American Council on Exercise (ACE). It's important to discuss with trainers your approach to eating. Many will have ideas other than those presented in this book. If your potential trainer objects to a very low-fat diet, for example, you can find another trainer.

Many other activities provide useful structures, too. For example, getting involved in community theater does not, at first blush, sound very active. Yet that involvement can get you out of the house and moving. More directly active recreational sports, like city league volleyball or softball, work great, as does joining a bowling league.

Join a Self-Help Group. This an excellent way to add structure and keep focused on your goals. There are two well-known and widely available self-help groups in the US and Canada, with a worldwide presence for Weight Watchers as well as online assistance:

- *Take Off Pounds Sensibly (TOPS).* Founded in 1948, TOPS has 200,000 members and 10,000 chapters operating in the US, Canada, and several other countries. To find the group meeting nearest you, go to www.tops.org, click on Meetings, and enter your zip code. I did this and found twenty-five, seven, and five chapters, respectively, within ten miles of several different locations I entered. Each chapter lists its meeting address and time, as well as the name of chapter leaders with phone numbers.
- TOPS focuses on self-monitoring, healthful eating, and staying active in a fashion consistent with the

principles of HOP. While TOPS may not advocate a very low-fat approach or the use of pedometers/Fitbits and the 12,000-step goal, it can still be very useful to keep you focused and motivated. The cost is also low. You will have to become a member and pay nominal chapter fees (each chapter sets its own fees to cover operating expenses).

These benefits outweigh the drawbacks of TOPS, which include the fact that some TOPS groups include people with substantial problems who can distract from the focus on the behaviors required for successful long-term weight control. TOPS group leaders also have minimal training.

- *Weight Watchers.* The only other non-professional approach that follows enough of the science of weight loss to warrant recommendation is Weight Watchers. Weight Watchers also encourages healthful eating and self-monitoring. There are over 20,000 Weight Watchers groups around the country. To find a meeting, go to www.weightwatchers.com and click on "Find a Meeting." Weight Watchers also provides an extensive and somewhat interactive online program, which is advertised heavily. However, research shows that actually attending group meetings produces much better results than the online program. Online programs simply do not engage participants very effectively, at least that's the case for the vast majority of people.

  Although Weight Watchers is famous for its "Points" program, Weight Watchers also offers a "Core Program" that doesn't use points, but rather focuses on self-monitoring, education, and support. Although very popular, the Weight Watchers point system fails the simplicity test—it's simply too complicated and over-emphasizes the importance of fiber. Weight controllers who attend Weight

Watchers meetings would be wise to remember that they won't benefit much from buying Weight Watchers products at these meetings. Just use the weekly meetings as an opportunity to improve your focus and commitment. Costs amount to about $10 per week. Other drawbacks: as with TOPS, the trainers receive minimal training and certainly are not professional therapists. Also, some members can prove distracting.

- *Other Self-help Approaches.* The other non-professional approaches, like Overeaters Anonymous, have numerous flaws in their approaches from a scientific perspective. I don't recommend any other non-professional approach aside from TOPS and Weight Watchers for this reason.

Get Help from a Professional

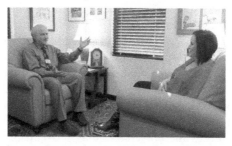

The above photo shows me talking with one of my colleagues, Heather Stokes, Georgia Pain and Spine Care's wonderful director of public and provider relations. Heather agreed to pretend to act like one of my clients for a story about my work in a local newspaper. Weight management service, when offered by a professional with my type of credentials, involves discussions that look like the one pictured here. We review self-monitoring records, discuss triumphs and challenges that happen every week, do constructive problem solving and planning, and keep the focus and accountability—and particularly the healthy obsession—thriving.

Some hospitals and medical centers offer professional weight management programs that can help some people achieve greater success than non-professional self-help programs. Look for programs directed by psychologists or other mental health professionals with expertise in cognitive-behavior therapy, the approach that has the best track record by far and forms the basis of much of this book. The better weight management programs are open-ended, providing help for unlimited periods of time, and definitely no less than one year. Longer-term programs tend to produce better outcomes.

The following three organizations also have listings of behavioral health professionals in virtually every area of the United States:

1. *Association for Behavioral and Cognitive Therapies* Go to www.abct.org and click on "Find a therapist."
2. *American Psychological Association* Go to www.apa.org and click on "Find a psychologist."
3. *National Association of Social Workers* Go to www.helpstartshere.org and click on "Find a social worker."

Calls to local hospitals and to psychology departments of local colleges and universities may prove helpful, too.

Immersion Programs. Programs like Wellspring immerse weight controllers in a structured world of healthy living and provide them with education, encouragement, and cognitive-behavior therapy to help them change. Some health spas provide the type of intensive experience that could result in rapid weight loss and build momentum to develop a healthy obsession. Participating in immersion programs can help you experience genuine success, and success really can breed more success. It's unfortunate that it is so challenging to compete with the biological and environmental challenges that resist weight loss. It's certainly possible that you may not be able to overcome these barriers, even with help from professionals dedicated to the same scientific principles as those described in this book. If this is the case, a scientifically based immersion program can make a huge difference. Immersion can also solidify and strengthen commitment.

Parting Thoughts

I hope you have found a way to tame the Stymie Beasts that have prevented you from moving forward with the important goal of long-term weight control. HOP can really make a difference in your quest, especially when those Stymie Beasts get put firmly in their place—out of your way! You learned the keys within HOP, including the development of major resolve in the form of a burgeoning healthy obsession—an obsession focused on a very low-fat diet, self-monitoring, and staying active. Here's another key: If you never give up on this quest, you can keep barriers at bay and live a healthier and happier life.

You deserve no less.

GLOSSARY OF ACRONYMS

CBT: **Cognitive Behavior Therapy**—According to the leading professional organization focused on CBT, the Association for Behavioral and Cognitive Therapy (ABCT, http://www.abct.org/Home/, within which I am a Fellow), "CBT is the term used for a group of psychological treatments that are based on scientific evidence. CBT is different from many other therapeutic approaches by focusing on the ways that a person's cognitions (i.e., thoughts), emotions, and behaviors are connected and affect one another. Because emotions, thoughts, and behaviors are all linked, CBT approaches allow for therapists to intervene at different points in the [thinking-feeling-behaving] cycle." Some of the common scientifically based techniques used in CBT are self-monitoring, problem solving, contingency management, stimulus control, cognitive restructuring, and stress management.

HOP: Healthy Obsession Pathway—Developing a healthy obsession is the most important aspect of the VLF HOP program, an overarching mission—not just a goal. *Healthy obsession is defined as a sustained preoccupation with the planning and execution of target behaviors to reach a healthy goal.* In the case of weight management, those target behaviors include a VLF diet, 100% self-monitoring, and 12,000 steps per day. The illustration on the next page shows how immersion programs work, producing rapid weight loss via self-regulated efforts, leading to lifestyle change after developing a very powerful healthy obsession.

Immersion-to-Lifestyle Change Model

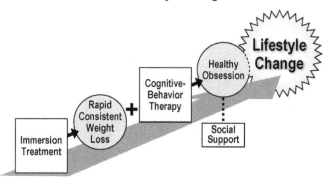

RET: Rational Emotive Therapy—RET is a technique originally developed by psychologist Dr. Albert Ellis in the mid-1950s. RET helps people identify the thoughts/beliefs that they use that can contribute to increased negative emotions (beliefs, for example, that use words like "should," "must," "have to," "always," "terrible," and "horrible"). RET encourages clients to change such beliefs (sometimes called "irrational beliefs" in RET or "unadaptive or problematic automatic thoughts") to those that emphasize greater degrees of choice in our actions and less dramatic/exaggerated potential for actions.

TUS: Therapeutic Understanding of Science—TUS is the use of scientifically sound information to make decisions and understand causes and effects.

VLF: Very Low-Fat—In nutritional science, VLF diets are those in which a person consumes 10% or fewer calories from fat per day. Targeting zero fat (and accepting 20 fatg at the most) helps most people achieve that very low fat goal. "Low-fat (LF)" diets have 11-19% calories from fat per day. Diets with 20-30% fat intake daily are considered "Moderate-fat (MF)" diets. 31% calories from fat and higher translates to a "High-fat (HF)" diet.

Aim for Zero Fat Grams

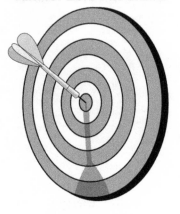

APPENDIX: FOOD SPECIFICS

For additional ideas and specific recipes, you can do an internet search using the phrases: "fat-free recipes" or "fat-free foods." Current examples from such searches include: http://www.fatfree.com/cgi-bin/recipes. cgi and http://www.eatingwell.com/recipes/18016/low-fat-fat-free/. The "Eating Well" website includes lots of reviews of each recipe; for example, thirty-eight reviews are posted for their "Slow-Cooker Moroccan Lentil Soup." This gives you great ideas, commentaries, and nearly an infinite possibility of likeable foods that like you too. I also co-wrote a cookbook with Carolyn Coulter (a supremely talented dietitian) of 188 very low-fat and amazingly good Wellspring recipes. It's only available on Amazon: https:// www.amazon.com/Wellspring-Weight-Loss-Cookbook-Fabulous/dp/1493740474/ref=sr_1_2?s=books&ie=UTF8 &qid=1510244558&sr=1-2&keywords=wellspring+weig ht+loss+cookbook.

Very Low-Fat Cooking

Here are a few very basic very low fat cooking tips:

MEATS
- Bake, broil, grill, or steam very lean meat, fish and poultry.
- Drain all fat
- Lean choices: fish, white meat chicken or turkey, 99% fat free ground turkey, pork tenderloin

- Fat free marinades (e.g., barbeque sauces; caribbean jerk; teriyaki; soy sauce variations) can tenderize and add flavor to chicken, very lean meats, and veggies.

VEGETABLES

- Stir fry vegetables in fat-free broth or light soy sauce.
- Add fat-free yogurt, sour cream, salsa,or honey mustards to white and sweet potatoes.
- Lemon/lime or pepper or chili or cajun powder can add interesting spice to veggies.
- Char-grill veggies

REFERENCES

Chapter 1–Introduction

Anderson, C.A., Miller, R.S., Riger, A.L., Dill, J.C., & Sediekes, C. (1994). Behavioral and characterological attributional styles as predictors of depression and loneliness: Review, refinement and test. *Journal of Personality and Social Psychology, 66,* 549-558.

Ellis, A., & Harper, R.A. (1975). *A new guide to rational living.* Hollywood, CA: Wilshire Book Co.

Frost, R.O., & Marten, P.A. (1990). Perfectionism and evaluative threat. *Cognitive Therapy and Research, 14,* 559-572.

Gilovich, T. Griffin, D. & Kahneman, D. (Eds.) (2002). *Heuristics and biases: The psychology of intuitive judgment.* NY: Cambridge University Press.

Kahneman, D. (2011). *Thinking fast and slow.* NY: Farrar, Straus and Giroux.

Kahneman, D., Slovic, P. & Tversky, A. (1982). *Judgment under uncertainty: Heuristics and biases.* NY: Cambridge University Press.

Schlenker, B.R., Pontari, B.A., & Christopher, A.N. (2001). Excuses and character: Personal and social implications of excuses. *Personality and Social Psychology Review, 5,* 15-32.

Tversky, A. & Kahneman, D. (1974). Judgment under uncertainty: Heuristics and biases. *Science, 185,* 1124-1131.

Chapter 2–Nature and Nurture of the Seven
Stymie Beasts

Bruner, J.S., & Postman, L. (1949). On the perception
of incongruity: A paradigm. *Journal of Personality, 18,*
206-223.

Gilovich, T. Griffin, D. & Kahneman, D. (Eds.)
(2002). *Heuristics and biases: The psychology of intuitive
judgment.* NY: Cambridge University Press.

Kahneman, D. (2011). *Thinking fast and slow.* NY:
Farrar, Straus and Giroux.

Kahneman, D., Slovic, P. & Tversky, A. (1982).
Judgment under uncertainty: Heuristics and biases. NY:
Cambridge University Press.

Kahneman, D., Frederickson, B.I., Schreiber, C.A., &
Redelmeier, D.A. (1993). When more pain is preferred to
less: Adding a better end. *Psychological Science, 4,* 401-405.

Katahn, M. (1989). *The t-factor diet.* NY: Norton Press.

Kirschenbaum, D.S., O'Connor, E.A., & Owens, D.
(1999). Positive illusions in golf: Empirical and conceptual
analyses. *Journal of Applied Sport Psychology, 11,* 1-27.

Kuhn, T.S. (1962). *The structure of scientific revolutions.*
Chicago, IL: The University of Chicago Press.

Lichtenstein, S., Slovic, P., Fischhoff, B., Layman, M.,
& Coombs, B. (1978). Judged frequency of lethal events.
*Journal of Experimental Psychology: Human Learning
and Memory, 4,* 551-578.

Slovic, P. Finucane, M., Peters, E. & MacGregor, D.C.
(2002). The affect heuristic. In T. Gilovich, D. Griffin,
& D. Kahneman, D. (Eds.) *Heuristics and biases: The
psychology of intuitive judgment,* pp.397-420. NY:
Cambridge University Press.

Taylor, S.E., & Brown, J.D. (1994). Positive illusions
and well-being: Separating fact from fiction. *Psychological
Bulletin, 11,* 21-27.

Tversky, A. & Kahneman, D. (1974). Judgment under
uncertainty: Heuristics and biases. *Science, 185,* 1124-1131.

Velanovich, V. (2000). Laparoscopic vs. open surgery: A preliminary comparison of quality-of-life outcomes. *Surgical Endoscopy,* 14, 16-21.

Chapter 3–Two Ways to Tame Your Stymie Beasts

Burns, D.E. (1989). *The feeling good handbook: Using the new mood therapy in everyday life.* NY: William Morrow & Company.

Davis, W. (2011). *Wheat belly.* NY: Rodale.

Dispirito, R. (2016). *The negative calorie diet.* NY: Harper Collins.

Fung, J. (2016). *The obesity code.* Vancouver, Canada: Greystone.

Gundry, S.R. (2008). *Dr. Gundry's diet evolution.* NY: Harmony/Random House.

Hartwig, D., & Hartwig, M. (2012). *It starts with food.* Las Vegas, NV: Victory Belt.

Hartwig, M., & Hartwig, D. (2015). *The whole 30.* NY: Houghton Mifflin Harcourt.

Hyman, M. (2016). *Eat fat, get thin.* NY: Little Brown.

Ellis, A., & Harper, R.A. (1975). *A new guide to rational living.* Hollywood, CA: Wilshire Book Co.

Hansen, C.J., Stevens, L.C., & Coast, J.R. (2001). Exercise duration and mood: How much is enough to feel better? *Health Psychology,* 20, 267-275.

Kirschenbaum, D. S. (2014). *Athlete, not food addict: Wellspring's seven steps to lose weight.* Far Hill, NJ: New Horizon Press.

Lent, M.R., Eichen, D.M., Goldbacher, E., Wadden, T.A., & Foster, G.D. (2014). Relationship of food addiction to weight loss and attrition during obesity treatment. *Obesity,* 22, 52-55.

Pomroy, H. (2012). *The fast metabolism diet.* NY: Harmony/Random House.

Poti, J.M., Mendez, M.A., Ng, W.W., & Popkin, B.M. (2105). Is the degree of food processing and convenience linked with the nutritional quality of foods purchased by

US households? *American Journal of Clinical Nutrition*, *99*, 1-12.

Schwarz, N., Strack, F., Hilton, D., & Naderer, G. (1991). Base rates, representativeness, and the logic of conversation: The contextual relevance of "irrelevant" information. *Social Cognition, 9*, 67-84.

Stork, T. (2016). *The lose your belly diet*. Los Angeles, CA: Ghost Mountain.

Vogel, L. (2017). *The keto diet*. Las Vegas, NV: Victory Belt.

Wadden, T.A. (1993). The treatment of obesity: An overview. In A.J. Stunkard & T.A. Wadden (Eds.), *Obesity: Theory and therapy (2nd Ed.)*, pp.197-218. NY: Raven Press.

Chapter 4–HOP Step 1: Understanding the Causes of Excess Weight

Bouchard, C., Tremblay, A., et al., (1990). The response to long-term overfeeding in identical twins. *New England Journal of Medicine, 322*, 1477-1482.

Brownell, K.D. & Horgen, K.B. (2004). *Food fight*. Chicago: Contemporary Books.

Costa, P.I., & McCrae, R.R. (1992). *Revised NEO Personality Inventory (NEO-PI-R) and NEO Five-Factor Inventory (NEO-FFI) professional manual*. Odessa, FL: Psychological Assessment Resources.

Goldberg, L.R. (1992). The development of markers for the big-five factor structure. *Psychological Assessment, 4*, 26-42.

Gosling, S.D., Rentfrow, P.J., & Swann, W.B. (2003). A very brief measure of the Big-Five personality domains. *Journal of Research in Personality, 37*, 504-528.

Hampson, S.E., Edmonds, G.W., Goldberg, L.R., Dubanoski, J.P., & Hillier, T.A. (2013). Childhood conscientiousness relates to objectively measured adult physical health four decades later. *Health Psychology, 32*, 925-928.

Hartigan, K.J., Baker-Strauch, D., & Morris, G.W. (1982). Perceptions of the causes of obesity and responsiveness to treatment. *Journal of Counseling Psychology, 29,* 478-485.

Johnson, W.G., & Wildman, H.E. (1983). Influence of external and covert food stimuli on insulin secretion in obese and normal persons. *Behavioral Neuroscience, 97,* 1025-1028.

Kelly, K.P., & Kirschenbaum, D.S. (2011). Immersion treatment for childhood and adolescent obesity: The first review of a promising intervention. *Obesity Reviews, 12,* 37-49.

Kirschenbaum, D.S. (2010). Weight loss camps in the US and the Immersion-to-Lifestyle Change model. *Childhood Obesity, 6,* 318-323.

Kirschenbaum, D.S., Craig, R.D., & Tjelmeland, L. (2007). *Sierra's weight-loss solution for teens and kids.* NY: penguin.

Kirschenbaum, D.S., & Gierut, K.J. (2013). Treatment of childhood and adolescent obesity: An integrative review of recent recommendations from five expert groups. *Journal of Consulting and Clinical Psychology, 81,* 347-360.

Lang, Peter J. (1995). The emotion probe: Studies of motivation and attention. *American Psychologist, 50,* 372-385.

McAdams, D.P., & Pals, J.L. (2006). A new big five: Fundamental principles for an integrative science of personality. *American Psychologist, 61,* 204-217.

Skelton, J. A., Goff, D. C., Ip, E., & Beech, B. M. (2011). Attrition in a multidisciplinary pediatric weight management clinic. *Childhood Obesity, 7,* 185–193.

Chapter 5–HOP Step 2: Developing a Healthy Obsession
Baker, R.C., & Kirschenbaum, D.S. (1993). Self-monitoring may be necessary for successful weight control. *Behavior Therapy, 24,* 377-394.

Baker, R.C., & Kirschenbaum, D.S. (1998). Weight control during the holidays: Highly consistent self-monitoring as a potentially useful coping mechanism. *Health Psychology, 17,* 367-370.

Barnard, N.D., Akhtar, A., & Nicholson, A. (1995). Factors that facilitate compliance to lower fat intake. *Archives of Family Medicine, 4,* 153-158.

Braet, C. & Van Winckel, M. (2000). Long-term follow-up of a cognitive behavioral treatment program for obese children. *Behavior Therapy, 31,* 55-74.

Baumeister, R.F., Heatherton, T.F., & Tice, D.M. (1994). *Losing control: How and why people fail at self-regulation.* San Diego, CA: Academic Press.

Bessesen, D.H., Rupp, C.L., & Eckel, R.H. (1995). Dietary fat is shunted away from oxidation, toward storage in obese Zucker rats. *Obesity Research, 3,* 179-189.

Boozer, C.N., Brasseur, A., & Atkinson, R.L. (1993). Dietary fat affects weight loss and adiposity during energy restriction in rats. *American Journal of Clinical Nutrition, 58,* 846-852.

Borushek, A. (2017). *The Calorie King calorie, fat and carbohydrate counter.* Huntington Beach, CA: Family Health Publications.

Boutelle, K.N., & Kirschenbaum, D.S. (1998). Further support for consistent self-monitoring as a vital component of successful weight control. *Obesity Research, 6,* 219-224.

Boutelle, K.N., Kirschenbaum, D.S., Baker, R.C., & Mitchell, M.E. (1999). How can obese weight controllers minimize weight gain during the high-risk holiday season? By self-monitoring very consistently. *Health Psychology, 18,* 364-368.

Campbell, T.C. with Campbell, T.M. (2005). *The China Study: Startling implications for diet, weight loss, and long-term health.* Dallas, TX: BenBella Books.

Caraher, K.J., & Kirschenbaum, D.S. (2014). "I see inspiration everywhere": Potential keys to nurturing healthy obsessions by very successful young weight controllers. *Childhood Obesity, 10,* 518-522.

Carver, C.S., & Scheier, M.F. (1990). Origins and functions of positive and negative affect: A control-process view. *Psychological Review, 97,* 19-35.

Ericsson, K.A., & Charness, N. (1994). Expert performance: Its structure and acquisition. *American Psychologist, 49,* 725-747.

Dobbing, J. (Ed.). (1987). *Sweetness.* NY: Springer-Verlag

Kirschenbaum, D.S. (1987). Self-regulatory failure: A review with clinical implications. *Clinical Psychology Review, 7,* 77-104.

Gately, P.J., Cooke, C.B., Butterly, R.J., Mackreth, P., & Carroll, S. (2000). The effects of a children's summer camp programme on weight loss, with a 10-month follow-up. *International Journal of Obesity, 24,* 1445-1453.

Gierut, K.J., Pecora, K.M., & Kirschenbaum, D.S. (2012). Highly successful weight control by formerly obese adolescents: A qualitative test of the healthy obsession model. *Childhood Obesity, 8,* 455-465.

Geiselman, P.J., & Novin, D. (1982). The role of carbohydrates in appetite, hunger and obesity. *Appetite, 3,* 203-223.

Harris, J.K., French, S.A., Jeffery, R.W., McGovern, P., & Wing, R.R. (1994). Dietary and physical activity correlates of long-term weight loss. *Obesity Research, 2,* 307-313.

Hensen, C.J., Stevens, L.C., & Coast, J.R. (2001). Exercise duration and mood state: How much is enough to feel better? *Health Psychology, 20 ,* 267-275.

Hill, J.O., Drougas, H., & Peters, J.C. (1993). Obesity treatment: Can diet composition play a role? *Annals of Internal Medicine, 119,* 694-697.

Israel, A.C., & Shapiro, L.S. (1985). Behavior problems of obese children enrolling in a weight reduction program. *Cognitive Therapy and Research, 6,* 451-460.

Jeffery, R.W., Hellerstedt, W.L., French, S.A. & Baxter, J.E. (1995). A randomized trial of counseling for fat restriction versus calorie restriction in the treatment of obesity. *International Journal of Obesity, 19,* 132-137.

Kanfer, F.H., & Karoly, P. (1972). Self-control: A behavioristic excursion into the lion's den. *Behavior Therapy, 3,* 398-416.

Kirschenbaum, D.S. (1987). Self-regulatory failure: A review with clinical implications. *Clinical Psychology Review, 7,* 77-104.

Kirschenbaum, D.S. (1994). *Weight loss through persistence: Making science work for you.* Oakland, CA: New Harbinger.

Kirschenbaum, D.S. (2000). *The 9 truths about weight loss.* NY: Holt.

Kirschenbaum, D.S. (2006) *The healthy obsession program: Smart weight loss instead of low-carb lunacy.* Dallas, TX: BenBella Books.

Kirschenbaum, D.S. (2014). *Athlete, not food addict.* Far Hills, NJ: New Horizon Press.

Kirschenbaum, D.S., Craig, R.D., Kelly, K.P., & Germann, J.N. (2007). Immersion programs for treating pediatric obesity: Follow-up evaluations of Wellspring Camps and Academy of the Sierras—a therapeutic boarding school. *Obesity Management, 3,* 261-266.

Kirschenbaum, D.S., Germann, J.N., & Rich, B.H. (2005). Treatment of morbid obesity in low-income minority adolescents: Participant and parental self-monitoring as determinants of initial success. *Obesity Research, 13,* 1527-1529.

Kirschenbaum, D.S., & Karoly, P. (1977). When self-regulation fails: Tests of some preliminary hypotheses.

Journal of Consulting and Clinical Psychology, 45, 1116-1125.

McGuire, M.T., Wing, R.R., Klem, M.L., Lang, W. & Hill, J.O. (1999). What predicts weight regain in a group of successful weight losers? *Journal of Consulting and Clinical Psychology, 67,* 177-185.

McGuire, M.T., Wing, R.R., Klem, M.L., & Hill, J.O. (1999). Behavioral strategies of individuals who have maintained long-term weight losses. *Obesity Research, 7,* 334-341.

Perri, M.G., Anton, S.D. et al. (2002). Adherence to exercise prescriptions: Effects of prescribing moderate versus higher levels of intensity and frequency. *Health Psychology, 21,* 452-458.

Perri, M.G., Nezu, A.M., & Viegener, B.J. (1992). *Improving the long-term management of obesity: Theory, research and clinical guidelines.* New York: John Wiley.

Schlundt, D.G., Sbrocco, T., & Bell, C. (1989). Identification of high risk situations in a behavioral weight loss program: Application of the relapse prevention model. *International Journal of Obesity, 13,* 223-234.

Sperduto, W.A., Thompson, H.S., & O'Brien, R.M. (1986). The effect of target behavior monitoring on weight loss and completion rate in a behavior modification program for weight reduction. *Addictive Behaviors, 11,* 337-340.

Stice E. (1998). Prospective relation of dieting behaviors to weight change in a community sample of adolescents. *Behavior Therapy, 29,* 277-297.

Subrahmanyam, K., Kraut, R.E., Greenfield, P.M., & Gross, E. F. (2000). The impact of home computer use on children's activities and development. *Children and Computer Technology, 10,* 123-140.

Wadden, T.A. (1993). Treatment of obesity by moderate and severe caloric restriction: Results of clinical research trials. *Annals of Internal Medicine, 119,* 688-693.

Weinberg, R.S. (1988). *The mental advantage: Developing your psychological skills in tennis.* Champaign, IL: Leisure Press.

Chapter 6—HOP Step 3: Eating to Lose

Agatston, A. (2003). *The South Beach diet: The delicious, doctor-designed, foolproof plan for fast and healthy weight loss.* Emmaus, PA: Rodale Press.

Atkins, R.C. (1998). *Dr. Atkins' New diet revolution.* New York, NY: Avon Books.

Barnard, N.D., Akhtar, A., & Nicholson, A. (1995). Factors that facilitate compliance to lower fat intake. *Archives of Family Medicine, 4,*153-158.

Bessesen, D.H., Rupp, C.L., & Eckel, R.H. (1995). Dietary fat is shunted away from oxidation, toward storage in obese Zucker rats. *Obesity Research, 3,*179-189.

Blackburn, G. L. The low-fat imperative. *Obesity, 16,* 5-6.

Borushek, A. (2017). *The CalorieKing calorie, fat and carbohydrate counter.* San Diego, CA: Family Health Publications.

Boozer, C.N., Brasseur, A., & Atkinson, R.L. (1993). Dietary fat affects weight loss and adiposity during energy restriction in rats. *American Journal of Clinical Nutrition, 58,* 846-852.

Campbell, T. C. (2005). *The China Study: Startling implications for diet, weight loss and long-term health.* Dallas, TX: BenBella Books.

Fleming, R.M. (2002). The effect of high-, moderate-, and low-fat diets on weight loss and cardiovascular disease risk factors. *Preventive Cardiology, 5,* 110-118.

Harris, J.K., French, S.A., Jeffery, R.W., McGovern, P., & Wing, R.R. (1994). Dietary and physical activity correlates of long-term weight loss. *Obesity Research, 2,* 307-313.

Hill, J.O., Drougas, H., & Peters, J.C. (1993). Obesity treatment: Can diet composition play a role? *Annals of Internal Medicine, 119,* 694-697.

Kaplan, H. et al. (2017). Coronary atherosclerosis in indigenous South American Tsimane: A cross-sectional cohort study. *Lancet, 389,* 1730-1739.

Kirschenbaum, D.S. (2005). Very low-fat diets are much better than low-carbohydrate diets: A position paper based on science. *Patient Care, 39,* 47-55.

Kirschenbaum, D.S. (2006) *The healthy obsession program: Smart weight loss instead of low-carb lunacy.* Dallas, TX: BenBella Books.

Kirschenbaum, D. S. (2014). *Athlete, not food addict: Wellspring's Seven Steps to Lose Weight.* Far Hill, NJ: New Horizon Press.

Mann, T., Tomiyana, A.J. et al. (2007). Medicare's search for effective obesity treatments: Diets are not the answer. *American Psychologist, 62,* 220-233.

Nachers, L.M., Middleton, K.R., Dubyak, P.J., Daniels, M.J., Anton, S.D., & Perri, M.G. (2013). Effects of prescribing 1,000 versus 1,500 kilocalories per day in the behavioral treatment of obesity: A randomized trial. *Obesity, 21,* 2481-2487.

Ornish, D. et al. (1998). Intensive lifestyle change for reversal of coronary heart disease. *JAMA, 280,* 2001-2007.

Rozin, P., Ashmore, M., & Markwith, M. (1996). Lay conceptions of nutrition: Dose insensitivity, categorical thinking, contagion, and the monotonic mind. *Health Psychology, 15,* 438-447.

Sears, B. & Lawren, B. (1995). *The zone: A dietary road map to lose weight permanently, reset your genetic code, prevent disease, achieve maximum physical performance.* New York, NY: HarperCollins.

Stice, E. (1998). Prospective relation of dieting behaviors to weight change in a community sample of adolescents. *Behavior Therapy, 29,* 277-297.

Van Horn, L., & Kavey, R.E. (1997). Diet and cardiovascular disease prevention: What works? *Annals of Behavioral Medicine, 19,*197-212.

Wadden, T.A., & Osei, S. (2002). The treatment of obesity: An overview. In T.A. Wadden & A.J. Stunkard (Eds.) *Handbook of obesity treatment* (pp.229-248). New York: Guilford Press.

Weigle, D.S., Cummings, D.E., et al. (2003). Roles of leptin and ghrelin in the loss of body weight caused by a low fat, high carbohydrate diet. *Journal of Clinical and Endocrinological Metabolism, 88,*1577-1586.

Chapter 7—HOP Step 4: Maximizing Movement

Andersen, R.E., Wadden, T.A., & Barlett, S. J. (1999). Effects of lifestyle activities versus structured aerobic exercise in obese women: A randomized trial. *JAMA, 281,* 335-340.

Baechle, T.R., & Groves, B.R. (1992). *Weight training: Steps to success.* Champaign, IL: Leisure Press.

Blair, S.N. (1991). *Living with exercise.* Dallas, TX: American Health Publishing Co.

Blair, S.N. (1991). Weight loss through physical activity. *Weight Control Digest, 1,* 17, 20-24.

Carpenter, R.A. (2004). Getting in step with counters. *Weight Management Newsletter of the American Dietetic Association, 1,* 1-2.

Curless, M.R. (1992). Only the fit stay young. *Self,* September, pp. 180-181.

Dishman, R.K. (Ed.). (1988). *Exercise adherence: Its impact on public health.* Champaign, IL: Human Kinetics Publishers.

Donahoe, C.P., Jr., Lin, D.H., Kirschenbaum, D.S., & Keesey, R.E. (1984). Metabolic consequences of dieting and exercise in the treatment of obesity. *Journal of Consulting and Clinical Psychology, 52,* 827-836.

Galvin, J. (1991). *The exercise habit: Your personal road map to developing a lifelong exercise commitment.* Champaign, IL: Human Kinetics Publishers.

Heil, J. (1993). *Psychology of sport injury.* Champaign, IL: Human Kinetics Publishers.

Kendzierski, D., and Johnson, W. (1993). Excuses, excuses, excuses: A cognitive behavioral approach to exercise implementation. *Journal of Sport and Exercise Psychology, 15,* 207-219.

Kusinitz, I., Fin, M., & Editors of Consumer Reports Books. (1983). *Physical fitness for practically everybody: The consumer's union report on exercise.* Mount Vernon: NY: Consumers Union.

Latella, F.S., Conkling, W., & Editors of Consumers Reports Books. (1989). *Get in shape stay in shape.* NY: Consumer Reports Books.

Rippe, J.M., & Amend, P. (1992). *The exercise exchange program.* NY: Simon & Schuster.

Vickery, S. & Moffat, M. (1999). *The American Physical Therapy Association book of body repair and maintenance.* NY: Owl Books.

Chapter 8—HOP Step 5: Creating a Supportive World Around You

Barlow, D.H., & Rapee, R.M. (1991). *Mastering stress: A lifestyle approach.* Dallas: American Health Publishing Company.

Bourne, E.J. (1990). *The anxiety and phobia workbook.* Oakland, CA: New Harbinger Publications, Inc.

Burns, D.E. (1989). *The feeling good handbook: Using the new mood therapy in everyday life.* NY: William Morrow & Company.

Cautela, J.R., & Groden, J. (1991). *Relaxation: A comprehensive manual for adults, children, and children with special needs.* Champaign, IL: Research Press.

Davis, M., Eshelman, E.R. and McKay, M. (1995). *The relaxation & stress reduction workbook (4th ed.).* Oakland, CA: New Harbinger Publications, Inc.

Kirschenbaum, D.S. (1997). *Mind matters: 7 steps to smarter sport performance.* Carmel, IN: Cooper Publishing Group.

McKay, M., and Fanning, P. (1993). *Time out from stress.* Oakland, CA: New Harbinger Publications, Inc.

Meichenbaum, D. (1985). *Stress inoculation training.* NY: Pergamon.

Paine, W.S. (1982) (Ed.). *Job stress and burnout.* Beverly Hills, CA: Sage Publications.

Smith, R.E., Smoll, F.L., & Curtis, B. (1979). Coach effectiveness training: A cognitive-behavioral approach to enhancing relationship skills in youth sport coaches. *Journal of Sport Psychology, 1, 59-75.*

Tubesing, N.L., & Tubesing, D.H. (1990). *Structured exercises in stress management.* (vols. 1-4). Duluth, MN: Whole Person Press.

Weinberg, R.S., & Gould, D. (2006). *Foundations of sport and exercise psychology,* Fourth Edition. Champaign, IL: Human Kinetics.

ABOUT THE AUTHOR
DANIEL KIRSCHENBAUM, PH.D., ABPP

D r. Kirschenbaum is Director of Behavioral Health within a thriving integrative pain management practice in metro-Atlanta, Georgia Pain and Spine Care: https://www.gapaincare.com. He is also Professor of Psychiatry & Behavioral Sciences at Northwestern University. The American Psychological Association (APA) awarded Dr. Kirschenbaum both Fellow and Diplomate statuses; he also served as president of APA's Division of Exercise and Sport Psychology. Dr. Kirschenbaum has provided invited addresses at professional conferences worldwide, received numerous grants for research, and consulted with many organizations (e.g., National Basketball Association; Ladies Professional Golf Association; US Olympic Committee; WebMD; National Academy of Sports Medicine; Weight Watchers). Dr. Kirschenbaum has published thirteen books and more than 140 book chapters and articles in scientific journals. He was also the Chief Program Officer (designer) and Clinical Director of Wellspring, a program of weight loss camps and boarding schools that became the leading provider of treatment services for overweight young people in the US for many years. The Board of Directors of the American Council on Exercise unanimously endorsed his book, *The Nine Truths about Weight Loss,* as "the best book ever written for the public on how to lose weight and keep it off."

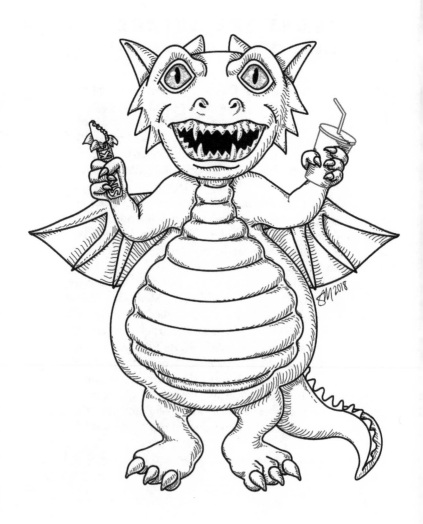

CPSIA information can be obtained
at www.ICGtesting.com
Printed in the USA
LVHW050015171118
597428LV00002B/2/P

9 781732 336254